The International Behavioural and Social Sciences Library

MENTAL HEALTH IN A CHANGING WORLD

TAVISTOCK

The International Behavioural and Social Sciences Library

MENTAL HEALTH
In 8 Volumes

I	Studies on Psychosis *Thomas Freeman*
II	Chronic Schizophrenia *Thomas Freeman, et al.*
III	Mental Illness in the Community *David Goldberg and Peter Huxley*
IV	Mental Illness in Childhood *V L Kahan*
V	Psychological Illness *E J R Primrose*
VI	Mental Health in a Changing World *Edited by Kenneth Soddy and Robert H Ahrenfeldt*
VII	Mental Health and Contemporary Thought *Edited by Kenneth Soddy and Robert H Ahrenfeldt*
VIII	Mental Health in the Service of the Community *Edited by Kenneth Soddy and Robert H Ahrenfeldt*

MENTAL HEALTH IN A CHANGING WORLD

Volume One of a Report on an International and Interprofessional Study Group convened by the World Federation for Mental Health

EDITED BY KENNETH SODDY
AND ROBERT H AHRENFELDT
WITH THE ASSISTANCE
OF MARY C KIDSON

Routledge
Taylor & Francis Group
LONDON AND NEW YORK

First published in 1965 by
Tavistock Publications Limited

Published in 2001 by
Routledge
2 Park Square, Milton Park, Abingdon, Oxfordshire OX14 4RN
711 Third Avenue, New York, NY 10017

First issued in paperback 2014

Routledge is an imprint of the Taylor and Francis Group, an informa business

British Library Cataloguing in Publication Data
A CIP catalogue record for this book
is available from the British Library

Mental Health in a Changing World
ISBN 0-415-26454-5
Mental Health: 8 Volumes
ISBN 0-415-26511-8
The International Behavioural and Social Sciences Library
112 Volumes
ISBN 0-415-25670-4

ISBN 13: 978-1-138-88139-6 (pbk)
ISBN 13: 978-0-415-26454-9 (hbk)

Mental Health in a Changing World

Volume I of a Report of an International and Interprofessional Study Group convened by the World Federation for Mental Health

Edited by KENNETH SODDY
and ROBERT H. AHRENFELDT
with the assistance of Mary C. Kidson

TAVISTOCK PUBLICATIONS
LONDON · SYDNEY · TORONTO · WELLINGTON

First published in 1965
by Tavistock Publications Limited
2 Park Square, Milton Park, Abingdon, Oxon, OX14 4RN
in 11 pt Plantin
by Butler & Tanner Ltd, Frome & London

To

JOHN RAWLINGS REES, C.B.E., M.D., F.R.C.P.,
this report in three volumes is affectionately
dedicated by the members of the
International Study Group
on Mental Health Perspectives, 1961

Volume I Mental Health in a Changing World
Volume II Mental Health and Contemporary Thought
Volume III Mental Health in the Service of the Community

Contents

Acknowledgements

Grateful acknowledgement is made to the National Institute of Mental Health, US Public Health Service, for US PHS Research Grant No. M-4998, which made it possible for the International Study Group to meet, for the summary report *Mental Health in International Perspective* to be prepared, and for editorial work on the current report in three volumes to be started; to the Grant Foundation of New York for bearing the cost of the salaries of the members of the Scientific Division of WFMH; to the Council for International Organizations of Medical Sciences for a subvention towards the preparation of resource materials; and to the WFMH US Committee Inc. for a grant towards the completion of the bibliography included in these volumes.

Obituary

ALBERT DEUTSCH died, suddenly and peacefully, in his sleep on Sunday, 18 June 1961, the seventh day in the work programme of the Study Group with which this Report is concerned. He was an experienced science writer and journalist, and perhaps the most distinguished 'communicator' in the field of mental health. His main assignment with the Study Group, in which he also took an active part, was to write the summary report for presentation at the International Congress on Mental Health in Paris, August–September 1961.

For thirty years Albert Deutsch had been completely dedicated to the task of raising the level of understanding in the United States of the problems of mental ill health, and made immense contributions to the promotion of awareness both of the need for change and of means towards its achievement.

Participants

The participants in the International Study Group came from eleven countries and represented fifteen fields of professional work. Their names, and their professional appointments at the time of the Study Group, are listed below:

DR H. C. RÜMKE (*Chairman*)
Professor of Psychiatry, University of Utrecht; Member, Royal Academy of Sciences in the Netherlands

DR ROBERT H. AHRENFELDT
Psychiatrist; Consultant and Research Associate, WFMH; *formerly* Dep. Asst Director of Army Psychiatry, War Office (UK)

THE REV. GEORGE C. ANDERSON
Director, Academy of Religion and Mental Health, New York

DR SIMON BIESHEUVEL
Director, National Institute for Personnel Research, South African Council for Scientific and Industrial Research, Johannesburg

†MR ALBERT DEUTSCH
Editor-in-Chief, *Encyclopaedia of Mental Health*, Washington, D.C.

DR JACK R. EWALT
Professor of Psychiatry, Harvard University Medical School; Superintendent, Massachusetts Mental Health Center; Director, Joint Commission on Mental Illness and Health, USA

DR RICHARD H. FOX
Psychiatrist, Bethlem Royal and Maudsley Hospitals; Hon. Asst Secretary, Research Committee, Mental Health Research Fund, UK; Secretary, Medical Research Council (UK) Sub-committee on Psychopathic Personality

PARTICIPANTS

DR FRANK FREMONT-SMITH

Director, Interdisciplinary Conference Program, American Institute of Biological Sciences; President and Chairman, Governing Board, WFMH US Committee Inc.; Co-Chairman, World Mental Health Year Committee

DR OTTO KLINEBERG

Professor and Chairman, Department of Social Psychology, Columbia University

DR DAVID M. LEVY

Lecturer in Psychiatry, College of Physicians and Surgeons, Columbia University; Consulting Psychiatrist, New York City Dept of Health; Visiting Professor of Psychiatry, Tulane University Medical School, New Orleans

DR TSUNG-YI LIN

Professor of Psychiatry, National Taiwan University Medical College, Taipei, Taiwan

DR STEPHEN A. MACKEITH

Consultant Psychiatrist and Physician Superintendent, Warlingham Park Hospital, Surrey; Adviser in Psychiatry to the County Borough of Croydon, Surrey; Consultant Psychiatrist, Mayday Hospital, Croydon

DR MARGARET MEAD

Visiting Professor of Anthropology, Menninger School of Psychiatry; Associate Curator of Ethnology, American Museum of Natural History; Adjunct Professor of Anthropology, Columbia University; Visiting Professor of Anthropology, School of Psychiatry, College of Medicine, University of Cincinnati

DR BEN S. MORRIS

Professor of Education and Director of the Institute of Education, University of Bristol

DR A. C. PACHECO E SILVA

Professor of Clinical Psychiatry, Faculty of Medicine, University of São Paulo, and School of Medicine of São Paulo; President, WFMH, 1960–61

DR JOHN R. REES

Director, WFMH

PARTICIPANTS

DR AASE G. SKARD

Associate Professor, Department of Child Psychology, University of Oslo

DR KENNETH SODDY

Scientific Director, WFMH; Physician and Lecturer in Child Psychiatry, University College Hospital and Medical School, University of London

DR GEORGE S. STEVENSON

Editor, *Mental Hygiene* (NAMH quarterly); President, WFMH, 1961–62; *formerly* National and International Consultant, NAMH; Medical Director, National Committee for Mental Hygiene, USA

DR ALAN STOLLER

Chief Clinical Officer, Mental Hygiene Authority, State of Victoria, Australia

DR MOTTRAM P. TORRE

Assistant Director, WFMH; Asst Attending Psychiatrist, St Luke's Hospital, New York

DR CLAUDE VEIL

Psychiatre de l'Association Interprofessionnelle des Centres Médicaux du Travail, Paris; Chargé de Conférences Techniques à l'Institut de Psychologie, Paris; Secrétaire du Groupe d'Hygiène Mentale Industrielle (Ligue d'Hygiène Mentale)

WHO Observers:

†DR E. EDUARDO KRAPF

Chief, Mental Health Section, WHO (*died 9 December 1963*)

DR DONALD F. BUCKLE

Regional Officer for Mental Health, WHO, Regional Office for Europe

DR TIGANI EL MAHI

Regional Adviser for Mental Health, WHO, Regional Office for the Eastern Mediterranean

Preface

It is with great pleasure that I have accepted the invitation to write a preface for the Report in three volumes of the International Study Group convened by the World Federation for Mental Health in 1961. For me, as Chairman of the Study Group, the reading of the manuscript has revived many memories of this fascinating meeting and stimulated a great number of thoughts. I believe that the report is of the greatest importance not only for those of us who had the good fortune to be members of the Study Group, but also for all those who are interested in both the scientific basis and the practice of mental health. In these restless and changing days, with their unending series of unpredictable international tensions, it may reasonably be asked whether it was worth while for a small group of men and women of widely varying individual scientific interests to come together in remote and lovely surroundings merely for the purpose of talking with each other. Although they had prepared working papers for the meeting and a number of references to the literature had been collected, they came without prepared scientific papers, 'official' documents, important statistical findings, films, or other concrete evidence, and also without an agreed conceptual foundation for the meeting. What they did bring with them was their experience of many and various forms of psychiatry, clinical and social psychology, sociology, education, or religion.

Within a prepared framework, which was designed more or less to cover the field of mental health, the Study Group spent its time in extempore discussion ranging over the oldest, the newest, and the most urgent problems of human beings. The conceptual aim of the conference was to provide an open exchange of thoughts, experiences, and views among a group of people of wide and varied experience, and by so doing to make a contribution to the science of man by the integration of the most diverse and highly specialized personal experience. The long-term hope was that the resulting synthesis of experience might make the sciences of man of greater value in the endeavour to improve mental health all over the world.

It is sometimes asked whether it is possible to achieve such ends by merely talking, and whether the not inconsiderable sums of money involved are well spent. Many of those who have been brought up in the natural science disciplines are not in sympathy with this type of programme. Natural scientists today are preoccupied with their attempts to raise the levels of methodological precision, to reach a higher level of objectivity, to clarify their models of thought, and to advance new hypotheses in the search for scientific principles. We can perfectly understand the point of view that the aims of the natural scientist as defined cannot be furthered by group discussion. On the other hand, we hope that many natural scientists are aware of the more intangible factors that appear to be operating in the field of the human mind, and of the relationships between people, and that they may be willing to agree that the special conditions obtaining in the field of mental health may require alternative and additional methods of approach.

We would ask the natural science purist who is unable to make any concession to a less pragmatic method of operation not to concern himself overmuch with these volumes. The purist is not likely to find a great deal of value in this Report. He will be distressed by a comparative lack of objectivity, and his scientific self-confidence may lead him into the detection of many errors. Above all, he will be greatly concerned by the lack of scientific proof for much that occupied the International Study Group's time.

Those who took part in the Study Group are fully convinced that such heterogeneous interprofessional and transcultural discussions are of high potential value, provided they are properly prepared and imaginatively planned. It is our conviction that this way of working enables us to arrive at the sources of new thinking. The work in which we are engaged in advancing the scientific knowledge of mental health is still only at its very beginning. The phase in which we are now working may fairly be called 'pre-scientific' – a necessary precursor of more objectively scientific ways of working. In our view, it is premature to narrow our interests to an exclusive specialization and search for objectivity. There is a place for both kinds of work – more concern with objectivity is urgently needed, but at the same time we need to preserve a view of the whole field in order to see more clearly the relative values of the many lines of specialized inquiry.

In this 'pre-scientific' era of mental health work, the primary need is to know how best to relate the many and various findings over the whole range of the field, at a time when much of the practical work that is being carried on is not of a highly specialized order. Major advances in conceptualization are not possible without the cooperation of a multidisciplined team. It has been said with some truth that from multidisciplined to undisciplined thinking is only one step. But, on the other hand, multidisciplinary thinking is the best defence against both the overestimation and the underestimation of the results of single-disciplined work. Only the multidisciplinary approach is likely to lead us to whole and basic truths.

This Report gives a number of perspectives over the whole of human life. Its subject-matter, which ranges widely around the world, will enrich the reader. The great complexity of the material and the diversity of thought may well have a confusing effect, but throughout the Report the connecting factor is the human being – Man as he is today in an ever-changing environment. If the reader is able to keep this connecting thread always in his mind, he will be at the same time surprised at the wide variety of human experience and fascinated by the essential sameness of human beings all over the world.

May I conclude by thanking, in the name of the members of the International Study Group, those who have completed the immense task of compiling these three volumes out of the many and various records of our discussions: Dr Kenneth Soddy, Dr Robert H. Ahrenfeldt, and Miss Mary C. Kidson.

Utrecht
January 1964

H. C. Rümke

Editors' Introduction

Mental Health in a Changing World is the first of three volumes that constitute the Report of the International Study Group on Mental Health, 1961, convened by the World Federation for Mental Health.

Volume I includes an account of the International Study Group, its background, composition, and work methods, as well as a summary of the major recommendations that the Group wished to make. The remainder of the volume is devoted to an account of the major developments and changes that have taken place transnationally in the field of mental health since the publication of the report of the International Preparatory Commission for the Third International Congress on Mental Health in London in 1948.

Volume II – *Mental Health and Contemporary Thought* – includes an account of the International Study Group's discussions on mental health in relation to the contemporary international scene, and on the light that these may throw on what is known about mental health. This account of the conceptual background is followed by a discussion concerning the training of professional people, and the information that educated members of the general public need in order to play a proper part in programmes of social action in this field.

Volume III – *Mental Health in the Service of the Community* – sets out the International Study Group's discussion of current diagnostic, therapeutic, and prophylactic action in the mental health field, and makes reference to the more salient aspects of research.

Originally conceived as one volume, the Report was divided into three volumes for the convenience of those readers who are concerned with a limited sector rather than the whole field of mental health. Like other aspects of social concern, the field of mental health action has widened very considerably in the last few decades. The editors believe that those whose main interest is in the promotion of mental health work may find Volume I the most absorbing of the three; those who are concerned with social problems and the light that the modern sciences of Man can throw on them may find Volume II more to their liking; and those who are engaged in direct therapeutic work, whether individual or community, may prefer Volume III. For the convenience of readers who do not wish to consult the complete set, the bibliography has been included in each of the volumes.

At the present time it is sometimes said that the method of conference discussion is out of fashion and that it can add little or nothing that is new to its subject. Those who set up the International Study Group on Mental Health, 1961, do not share this view; they consider that the conference discussion has fallen out of favour only among those people who have not understood either its full potentialities or the technical requirements for success. It is readily conceded that a conference may be useless, even harmful, if it is not properly prepared for, and if there is no clear idea of the aims; and, indeed, there is far more to a conference than the mere gathering together of people to talk about a subject. In this volume we have discussed some of the difficulties of people currently engaged in mental health work, and have emphasized the necessity for applying insights gained from modern psychology and allied sciences to the work problems involved. This is true of conferences no less than of other aspects of the work. It would not be reasonable, today, to convene a conference on a mental health subject without bringing to it all the insights available from studies of group dynamics.

It is well recognized that intercommunication is achieved most easily in a group that is homogeneous in terms of age, nationality or culture, educational level, and so on; and with the greatest difficulty when the group is markedly heterogeneous. The International Study Group, 1961, was, by design, interprofessional, transnational, and included a wide age-range. Without a considerable degree of heterogeneity, a study group on transnational mental health questions would be pointless. The inherent difficulties of heterogeneity were, we believe, successfully offset by the specific experience of the Study Group members. The nucleus around which the Study Group was formed was the Scientific Committee of the Federation, the members of which had been in the habit of meeting regularly over a period of about six years for the purpose of studying and writing reports on emerging mental health topics. This group was highly practised in intercommunication; and those members of the International Study Group who were not on the Scientific Committee, though not so closely organized at the outset, also brought with them a wealth of experience of communication across cultural and professional frontiers, and in every case were well known professionally to one or more members of the Scientific Committee.

Thus the Study Group, though apparently heterogeneous, and though coming from many different professions and nations, had in fact achieved a degree of homogeneity of interest in the mental health field before it started its work. The effect of this was quickly visible in the highly integrated work that the Study Group was able to accomplish within a period of two weeks.

Editors of reports are faced with the difficult choice of how far to reproduce verbatim records of discussions and how far to attempt to make a distillate. In the present instance we have tried to achieve a compromise between the extremes. Tape recordings were made of the entire discussions and, in addition, the members themselves had provided a number of working papers and annotations for the editors to draw upon. The main task of the editors has been to arrange the discussions in what appeared to them to be the most logical order, and then to write a considered commentary on the material, illustrating it where appropriate with extracts from the tape recordings and working papers.

The members of the Study Group have voluntarily accepted a group responsibility for what is written in these three volumes. Every member of the Group has had an opportunity to read and comment on the draft and, as far as possible, all the comments received have been acted upon by the editors. That these three volumes represent the agreed Report of the twenty-four members of the Study Group is true in spirit rather than in detail. It is not conceivable that every member agrees with every word that has been written, and in some instances the areas of individual disagreement may be quite wide. Wherever a known area of disagreement or open controversy has been touched upon in the text the editors have attempted to make this clear to the reader.

The editors have been at pains to ensure that the extensive bibliography is accurate and complete up to the summer of 1962. A few books published since that time have been brought to our notice and we have included these under the heading 'Supplementary Titles' but we lacked the facilities to ensure that the list of recent additions is complete.

The editors wish to record their very deep indebtedness to all the members of the Study Group, who have responded so willingly and generously to all requests made for working papers and for criticism and comments on the draft of this Report. A great deal of work has been put into these volumes by a large number of people. We are, of course, most particularly indebted to our Chairman, Professor Dr H. C. Rümke, for his guiding hand throughout the operation and for his highly valued contributions to the compilation of the Report.

We should like to add our own personal note of gratitude to our Editorial Assistant, Miss Mary Kidson, for her immense help throughout, and especially in organizing the very complex material in the later stages of report writing. To her name we would add the names of Miss Elizabeth Barnes, for providing a framework for the first draft of the Report, and Mr Peter Robinson, for his invaluable assistance with the bibliography.

We have found the compilation of this Report a most stimulating and extending experience, and we hope that it will give the reader some notion of the rich field of work to be found in mental health all over the world today.

London KENNETH SODDY
January 1964 ROBERT H. AHRENFELDT

PART ONE

The International Study Group 12–24 June 1961

I

Background to the Study Group

The International Study Group on Mental Health, 1961, was the direct successor of the International Preparatory Commission of 1948 that preceded the Third International Congress on Mental Health in London, August 1948. The 1948 Commission resulted in the publication of *Mental Health and World Citizenship* (12), which was presented to the London Congress a few weeks later; and it is tempting to draw a further parallel between 1948 and 1961 and point out that the summary report of the 1961 Study Group, entitled *Mental Health in International Perspective*, was presented to the Sixth International Congress on Mental Health in Paris, August 1961.

Closer examination of the historical facts suggests that the parallel between 1948 and 1961 is more apparent than real, that the 1961 meeting may be better regarded as an organic evolution from the 1948 Commission. During the intervening thirteen years world conditions and the shape of mental health work crossing national and cultural boundaries had changed enormously.

The great London Congress of 1948 was the occasion of the rebirth of international cooperation in the field of mental health after the disastrous years of war. The Congress did no more than mark the occasion, for the reopening of communications had mainly resulted from the farsightedness of Dr J. R. Rees and his colleagues.

International mental health work owes its origin to the late Clifford W. Beers and a small group of colleagues who, through the International Committee, provided the link between the First and Second International Congresses on Mental Health in Washington, 1930, and Paris, 1937, respectively. The Third Congress was unfortunately prevented by the second world war from meeting in Rio de Janeiro in 1941. However, although the war had destroyed all active international mental health cooperation, it also had the effect, paradoxically, when fighting ceased, of facilitating communication between leading figures in mental health work on both sides of the Atlantic, as they engaged in the immediate tasks of postwar social reconstruction.

It was Rees who had the vision in 1946 to realize that there existed an enormous potential for goodwill all over the world. He had the creative imagination to make use of the potential lines of communication which had opened up, to form small working parties with the object over a period of about two years of preparing material for the London Congress. These Preparatory Commissions, as they were termed, brought together about five thousand men and women of varying professions in small study groups, located in some twenty-seven countries. Their reports were collated during the summer of 1948 by a team of voluntary editors and were presented to the International Preparatory Commission which met at Roffey Park, Horsham, England. This International Commission was composed of twenty-five people who met over a period of sixteen days, and its report, entitled *Mental Health and World Citizenship* (12), which was presented to the Third International Congress on Mental Health, has become a classic.

The 1948 London Congress had a far-reaching effect on the field of mental health in enabling people the world over to communicate with each other once again, after the total deprivation of the war years. Its most practical contribution was the formation of the World Federation for Mental Health, which in its early days enjoyed the very great advantage of being able to build upon the work and goodwill of the Preparatory Commissions. To the newly formed body, *Mental Health and World Citizenship* represented an epitome of the best transcultural thought in the field of mental health, and it was extensively used as a source of ideas for the development of the work.

Ten years later the question of a new International Commission to review the state of mental health work began to be debated. The usefulness of *Mental Health and World Citizenship* had encouraged the idea that it would be most valuable to carry out a review, by a transnational and cross-disciplinary group, of the state of mental health action throughout the world and of the degree to which the recommendations in *Mental Health and World Citizenship* had been implemented. At the same time, the view was emerging that the 1948 statement, although by no means merely a topical or ephemeral document, was no longer representative of the main interests and emphases in the mental health field during the late 1950s. In 1948, when the world was painfully beginning to recover from the disasters of World War II, the question of international relations and the responsibility of each individual for humanity as a whole were perhaps the most burning of all mental health concerns. In 1958 the main emphasis appeared to be different, but at the time it was far from clear where the emphasis lay.

The considerable impetus given to mental health work everywhere by World Mental Health Year, 1960, provided a favourable opportunity for carrying out the long-cherished plan of the World Federation for Mental Health to repeat the International Preparatory Commission of 1948, but in terms of current problems. At first it was proposed that the new Commission should study the 1948 statement, rewrite it in terms of more currently topical problems, and make an evaluation of what had been achieved in implementing its recommendations. However, the early preparatory work for the new study group revealed that the emphasis in mental health work in many parts of the world had changed to such an extent that it would be better to leave the 1948 statement to stand as a landmark of progress. The International Study Group of 1961, therefore, was set up in order to make a fresh review of mental health activities throughout the world, to attempt to assess the significance of trends and developments, and to suggest new and promising lines for the future.

The World Federation for Mental Health has acknowledged its indebtedness to the United States National Institute of

Mental Health for bearing practically the whole of the cost of the meeting; to the Grant Foundation of New York for paying for the work of the then Scientific Director and his Technical Assistant, which made it possible for the preparatory work and organization and much of the editorial work of the Study Group to be undertaken; to the Council for International Organizations of Medical Sciences for its subvention to enable Dr Robert H. Ahrenfeldt to start on the collection and collation of preparatory material, six months before the date of the International Study Group; and to the WFMH US Committee Inc. for its grant to enable him to continue the bibliography for these volumes. The Federation's deep gratitude is due also to the Adèle Levy Foundation for being willing to underwrite the whole cost of the Study Group project until such time as financial support had become assured – a generous and considerate action that gave sufficient security to enable the preparations to be undertaken early enough to be effective.

SOURCE MATERIAL

Dr Ahrenfeldt began his preparatory work by passing the following sources of information rapidly under review:

WFMH publications:[1] books, cross-cultural studies, *World Mental Health* articles, WFMH Clearing House information and reports from Member Associations about work in their own countries; reports by various governments to the Sixth International Congress on Mental Health in Paris (August–September 1961), including reports on mental health services and programmes in Australia and Thailand by Dr Alan Stoller, and in Liberia by Dr Nathan Kline; reports by the Director of WFMH on visits to the Far East, Australasia, Central Africa, Central and South America, and by Professor Sivadon on his visit to Turkey.

UN agency reports, including WHO Expert Committee and Study Group reports and Technical Monographs; reports made avail-

[1] Full references to all material used in the text may be found in the bibliography.

able by the WHO Mental Health Section, Geneva, and the Mental Health Officers of WHO Regional Offices; WHO Mental Health Consultant visit reports, including three on Yugoslavia by Dr Tredgold, and others on Egypt by Dr Kraus, on North African countries by Dr Tigani el Mahi, on Israel by Dr Sunier, on Italy by Dr Lemkau, and on Greece by Dr Repond; various UNESCO Conferences on Education, including *Education and Mental Health* (1955), and the two-yearly survey of educational advances throughout the world; and the UN Social Commission report on *The World Social Situation.*

Report of the Joint Commission on Mental Illness and Health, New York.

Reports on mental health legislation: a survey by WHO; mental health legislation in the UK and Belgium; a comparison of the recommendations of *Neurosis and the Mental Health Services* (Blacker, 1946) with successive UK Ministry of Health (Board of Control) reports; reports by the NIMH (USA); and a survey compiled by Albert Deutsch.

Reports of non-governmental organizations: an American Psychiatric Association report on Costa Rica; the International Union of Child Welfare inquiry during World Mental Health Year into progress in child welfare.

Reviews of advances in psychiatry published in the *Journal of Mental Science* and the *American Journal of Psychiatry.*

Time permitted only a bird's-eye view of the vast array of books and articles on mental health published in medical, psychological, and sociological journals. Information on research projects was kindly supplied by the Bio-Sciences Exchange, Washington. The bibliographical bulletin on mental health compiled by Professor Carlos Nassar, University of Chile; the US Department of Health, Education, and Welfare bulletin on research relating to children; *Excerpta Medica*; Psychological and Social Science Abstracts; and the WHO, UNESCO, and ILO libraries and documentation were consulted.

The general aim with the preparatory material was to compile a series of syntheses of the relevant studies, including abstracts of the more significant material. The syntheses were reproduced and distributed in advance to the Study Group participants, together with detailed references to the source material.

In order to give the reader some idea of the complexity and extent of the field of modern mental health action, the guide that was drawn up for the organization of the preparatory material is given below. It was not anticipated that significant new material would be found in all of the specific areas mentioned, and, indeed, had this been so, the Study Group would have been overwhelmed with the weight of material. The review was planned exhaustively in order to gain an idea not only of what is going on but also of what is being neglected at the present time. It enabled the field of discussion of the Study Group to be reduced to a more manageable size by focusing attention only on those areas where significant advances had been made in the last decade or so, noting also where the major gaps occurred.

The preparatory material was organized in eight major sections and, where relevant, was separately scrutinized in respect of children, adolescents, adults, and the aged.

I *Clinical*

Recognition of disorder, and diagnosis
Recognition of social and cultural factors
Psychiatric hospitals and the community
Early consultation
The process of hospitalization
Inpatient work:
- the hospital as a therapeutic community
- day hospitals, night hospitals
- hospital techniques – open wards, pharmacology, and biochemistry
- medical therapy, shock therapy, etc.
- individual and group psychotherapy and psycho-analysis
- community, occupational, and recreational therapy

the senile patient
hospitals and patients' families
teamwork in hospital

Rehabilitation, after-care, social clubs, etc.
Outpatient work:
outpatients' departments of psychiatric hospitals
psychiatric outpatients' departments of general hospitals
the independent psychiatric clinic

The psychiatric wing of a general hospital
Special problems of children and adolescents:
developmental disorders
education, vocational guidance, and training
retardation, delinquency

2 *Research*

Epidemiology of mental disorder
Epidemiology of pathological behaviour
Studies in aetiology and pathology
Research into therapeutic methods
Follow-up studies
Child development studies in many cultures
Studies of vulnerable states in human life
Studies of human relationship formation in various cultures
Studies of factors promoting stability and psychological strength in various cultures

3 *Prophylaxis*

Measures intended to prevent psychiatric disorder:
encouragement of early consultation
role of the general practitioner
counselling services, marriage guidance
role of child guidance clinics in prevention
school psychological services
anti-addiction measures (alcohol, drugs, etc.)

Measures taken against factors considered to be significant in causation of psychiatric disorder:

- services to promote good family relationships
- support of parents of young children:
  - psychological counselling in child welfare services
  - paediatrician and public health nurse
  - parent education
  - mental health propaganda (see also public education)
- vocational guidance
- social protection of young children:
  - prevention of family breakdown
  - prevention of separation of babies and toddlers from their mothers
  - substitute care for separated children
  - adoption, fostering of children
- prophylaxis of malnutrition and deficiency diseases

Eugenic measures

4 *Professional Training*

Specialist training of psychiatrists, psychiatric nurses, psychiatric social workers, clinical psychologists, and non-medical psychotherapists

Psychotherapy by general medical practitioners

Mental health training, and training in teamwork and interprofessional cooperation, of:

- general practitioners, public health doctors, paediatricians, other medical, surgical, and gynaecological specialists, and medical undergraduates
- hospital, public health, and industrial nurses
- medical and general social workers
- educationalists

Mental health training of other professional personnel dealing with people:

- ministers of religion
- judges and lawyers

police, probation officers, and prison officers
military officers
industrial managements and foremen
social welfare and child care workers
politicians, local government officials, and diplomats

Maintenance of balance between the above training measures and the general state of public education about mental health

5 *Public Education in Mental Health*

Mass media:
press, films, radio and television, public meetings
Lecture courses, study groups, etc.

Parent education
Exhibitions and public advertisement
Pamphlets, posters, cartoons, film strips
Display methods in public health clinics, etc.
Distribution of regular bulletins on mental health topics (e.g. the *Pierre the Pelican* (Louisiana) series for parents of new babies)
Counselling, advice bureaux, etc.
The timing of public education in relation to individual and group needs

6 *Mental Health Implications in Other Fields of Science and Professional Practice*

Mental health principles and:
general hospital practice
general medical practice
public health practice
education – from nursery school to university
special education of handicapped children
care of children deprived of normal family life
the field of criminality and treatment of offenders
man management in industry and commerce
accidents and accident prevention

The impact of a psychiatric department on a general hospital

7 *Mental Health Implications in Social and Community Life*

Popular attitudes towards psychiatry, mental disorder, and deviant behaviour

Attitudes in the community towards psychiatric consultation

Prejudice within the community

Problems of bureaucracy and bureaucratic attitudes

The relationship between socio-economic security (including community welfare programmes) and mental health

Problems of community leadership in the absence of an educated cadre

Problems of changing attitudes:

- to sexuality
- to concepts of honesty, dishonesty, and delinquency
- to relations between young and old (including the concept of each by the other)
- to death and dying

Problems arising out of improvements of medical techniques:

- improved ability to detect the existence of subclinical disease (e.g. a primary tubercular focus)
- the preservation of the life of severely handicapped children
- reanimation (i.e. life preserved by artificial means (iron lung, and so on))

Mental health aspects of birth control, artificial insemination, euthanasia, sterilization, and therapeutic abortion

Mental health aspects of industrialization, population movements, automation, leisure, atomic energy; acceptance of refugees; retirement

Mental health aspects of community planning, new towns, etc.

8 *Mental Health and Cultural Attitudes*

Problems of cross-cultural communication, including cooperation between nations, transcultural prejudice, selection and training of personnel for transcultural work

Attitudes to and concepts of mental health promoted by different religions and ideologies

Cultural attitudes to psychiatric disorder, illness and death, sexuality
Cultural attitudes to fate, stress, anxiety, tension, suffering; and modes of release of tension
Comparisons of child-rearing practices, food habits, patterns of authority, family structure and function, qualities of interpersonal relationships, and their bearing upon the mental health of, and the concepts of mental health held in, society.

This guide demonstrates the fantastic complexity of the field of concern and activity that is nowadays embraced by the term 'mental health'. It should be re-emphasized that this scrutiny of preparatory material was in no sense an attempt to review progress, which would have been a mammoth undertaking occupying a number of years. The Study Group was concerned only with what was new and important.

Shortly before the Study Group met together, the preparatory material compiled by Dr Ahrenfeldt was circulated to each member, under the general heading of 'Critical Notes on Some Mental Health Problems and Activities in Recent Years', in the following areas:

1 Clinical aspects of mental health activities (administrative and clinical activities, and trends in planning and developing community mental health services)
2 Research
3 Prophylaxis
4 Mental health implications in other fields of medical practice, in education, the social sciences, and industry
5 Mental health in social and community life; and in relation to cultural attitudes.

The provisional bibliography that was issued, referring to each of these areas, included 372 titles.

We were grateful to receive in time for distribution at the Study Group an article by Dr E. E. Krapf and Mrs Joy Moser on 'Changes of Emphasis and Accomplishments in Mental Health

Work over the Last Twelve Years' (subsequently published in *Mental Hygiene* (5)); an article by Dr Donald F. Buckle on 'European Developments in Mental Health Practice'; and the 1960 report of the Regional Director of the Eastern Mediterranean Region of WHO on 'Mental Health'.

The following publications were selected, from among many that were suitable, as being of particular relevance to the Study Group, and were circulated to members in advance:

DUHL, LEONARD J.	Alcoholism: The Public Health Approach (296)
FERGUSON, R. S.	Side-effects of Community Care (136)
FREMONT-SMITH, F.	The Interdisciplinary Conference (55)
GEBER, M. & DEAN, R. F. A.	Psychological Factors in the Aetiology of Kwashiorkor (271)
KRAPF, E. E.	On the Pathogenesis of Epileptic and Hysterical Seizures (332)
KRAPF, E. E.	The International Approach to the Problems of Mental Health (3)
KRAPF, E. E.	The Work of the World Health Organization in the Field of Mental Health (4)
LECONTE, MAURICE	De la nécessité de tirer quelques enseignements de l'actualité de la criminalité psychiatrique révélée par la presse (476)
LINDSAY, T. F.	When Scientists stop being Human (659)
LIN, TSUNG-YI	Evolution of Mental Health Programmes in Taiwan (97)
MOSSE, HILDE L.	The Misuse of the Diagnosis, Childhood Schizophrenia (276)
RUHE, D. S. *et al.*	Television in the Teaching of Psychiatry (622)
SANDS, S. L.	Discharges from Mental Hospitals (178)
SODDY, K. (ed.)	Identity; Mental Health and Value Systems (40, 41)
WITTKOWER, E. D. & FRIED, J	A Cross-cultural Approach to Mental Health Problems (565)

ILO	Ergonomics: the Scientific Approach to Making Work Human (525)
ILO	Some Aspects of the International Migration of Families (544)
WFMH	*Mental Health and World Citizenship* (12)
WFMH	*Africa: Social Change and Mental Health* (493)
WFMH	*A Brief Record of Eleven Years, 1948–1959, and World Mental Health Year 1960* (20)
WHO	Technical Report: Programme Development in the Mental Health Field (391)
WHO	Suggested Outline for use in discussing 'Mental Health Programmes in Public Health Planning' (for 1962 World Health Assembly—unpublished)
WHO REGIONAL OFFICE FOR EUROPE	The Education of the Public in Mental Health Principles (Conference on Mental Hygiene Practice, Helsinki, 1959) (635)

Finally, each participant was invited to prepare some notes on a subject central to his or her own interest, for prior distribution as a working paper to other members of the Study Group. Since this had been largely an informal request, the Study Group itself decided that the working papers would not be published separately but, instead, would be used to illustrate the present volume.

The titles of the participants' working papers that were distributed are as follows:

Mental Health Concepts in Different Places

The Mental Health Association and the Moving Target of Cultural Difference and Cultural Change – change of role concepts and value orientations

Mental Health Work in Cross-cultural Situations, with special reference to underdeveloped areas.

Current Progress in the Mental Health Field in the United States of America

Problems of Mental Health in Latin America

Adaptations to Rapid Social Change in Southern Africa

Mental Health and International Service

Industrialization

The Place of Religion in Mental Health

Psychodynamics of Segregation

Perspectives in Social Psychiatry

The Intimate Role of the Family in Prophylaxis – notes on the strengthening, as opposed to traumatic, experiences of childhood

More Research is Desirable (in child guidance work)

Education and Mental Health

2

The Work of the Study Group

MEMBERSHIP

The members of the Study Group, with the exception of three members of WHO staff, were invited to attend in a personal and not a representative capacity. The main criteria adopted for the selection of members were:

To secure
1 a spread of professional disciplines
2 the widest possible range of cultures

To invite only those
3 who had had a wide experience of mental health work
4 who had made outstanding original contributions
5 who were experienced and able in communicating across professional, linguistic, and cultural boundaries.

The task of selection, difficult in any circumstances, was therefore greatly complicated by the five separate ranges of criteria that had to be considered. It is axiomatic that any individuals who fulfilled all the criteria of selection would already be more than fully loaded with work precisely because of their experience and gifts. Each intending participant in the Study Group had to be prepared to devote time to reading voluminous preparatory material, to travel and to spend two full weeks at the residential Study Group, and to take a hand in editing and criticizing the subsequent publications. It is a measure of the interest that the Study Group aroused and of the recognition of its importance that those few of the original list of persons to be invited who could not participate were unable to do so only because of previously arranged commitments.

A Steering Committee of three members was set up to select

participants for invitation. After a preliminary examination of the field, it was agreed that it was hopeless to attempt to follow any kind of representative principle. It is inconceivable that any twenty-five people could adequately represent all the professional disciplines concerned with mental health and, in addition, all cultures. The problem was hardly one of selection, but rather of the elimination of all but twenty-five of the many hundreds of people who have been working in the field of mental health in recent years and who could make a distinguished contribution to a Study Group. As a first step in the elimination process it was agreed, since the Study Group was a WFMH occasion, to consider only those who had shown some awareness of and a constructive attitude towards the Federation during the previous twelve years, and who had a record of active work in the international field. As indicated above, with more than forty countries represented among the membership of WFMH and at least fifteen distinctive professional disciplines to be considered, no kind of quota system could be applied to the filling of a mere twenty-five places. Another complication was that of language. It is an important WFMH principle that all people, whatever their language, should have full opportunity to contribute to international mental health work, but it is none the less inescapable that a multiplicity of languages adds enormously to the technical problems and cost of a meeting, and also makes the whole task of effective intercommunication very much more complex. In the end, it was decided to use only English and French, which regrettably cut down the width and spontaneity of contribution, but the practical arguments in favour of this decision could not be challenged.

It is interesting to note that the twenty-six participants in the International Preparatory Commission of 1948 were drawn from seven professional disciplines and ten different countries. In the Introduction to *Mental Health and World Citizenship* (12) it is stated that the members of the Commission had had an exceptionally rich experience within the broad categories of their own professions and that many of them had worked in borderline areas, in cooperation with other professions. It was thought that 'this group was composed of men and women of broad outlook and background'.

The twenty-five participants in the International Study Group, 1961, were drawn from some thirteen distinct professional disciplines and from eleven countries. The increase in the number of disciplines represented in the Group was due in part to the greater professional differentiation that had taken place in the intervening thirteen years. The rigid categories of the established professions are tending to break down into a number of newly recognized groups, e.g. the psychiatrist in public health practice, in which area the 1961 Study Group was strongly represented. The Group also included a minister of religion in his capacity as such (the 1948 Commission had included a priest in his capacity as a psychologist), and another new addition was that of a professional science writer who had been entrusted with the compilation of the first summary report of the Study Group for presentation to the Sixth International Congress on Mental Health in Paris, August 1961.

LOCAL ARRANGEMENTS

Some readers will be interested in the practical problems of conducting international meetings, as illustrated by the brief description that follows.

The International Study Group was in continuous session from 12 to 24 June inclusive, at the conference centre, Roffey Park, near Horsham, Sussex. This conference centre was designed for small group meetings and comprises twenty-five bedrooms, three lounges or meeting rooms and a bar situated in the dormitory block, a dining room and kitchen at about one hundred yards' distance, and a conference room and office suite about half a mile away. The whole is set in the beautiful grounds of two contiguous country houses, converted for use as an Industrial Rehabilitation Centre.

For a group of twenty-five people, this style of accommodation is very pleasant during the summer, provided that the weather is reasonably fine, which is always problematical in the English climate. The walk to and from the conference room four times a day was much enjoyed by the more able-bodied members of the party, but a minibus more than justified its hire by the convenience that it afforded.

The great practical disadvantage of the facilities at Roffey Park was that sleeping accommodation was not available for the three members of the secretarial staff, the précis writer, and the two interpreters. The experience of many small international meetings has shown that it is highly advantageous to have all the members of the group, whatever their role, living together and sharing in the community life. The administrators, the interpreters, and those who compile the records make a very material and important contribution to the whole work of the group and they give best value if they are included as full members. In the present case, overflow accommodation was secured at hotels at Horsham, four miles away, and transport was provided morning and evening. The staff concerned were encouraged to take a full part in all the social and recreational activities of the group.

Discussions were conducted in English and French, with simultaneous interpretation. Members whose first language was neither of these were asked to select whichever of the two languages they knew best, and not to attempt English just because the majority happened to be English- rather than French-speakers.

THE WORK PLAN

In order to make a start on the morning of Monday, 12 June, the Study Group convened on the evening of 11 June so that initial contact would be at a social level. Although the majority of members were already acquainted with each other, there were some who were comparative strangers to the rest. Unfortunately, illness at the last moment prevented the attendance of Dr Solange Faladé, a French-trained anthropologist from West Africa. It was too late to find a replacement who would give a similar cultural and professional representation, but the Study Group was fortunate in securing, without previous notice, the attendance of Dr Richard Fox, a psychiatrist of the United Kingdom.

At the opening session on the morning of Monday, 12 June, the Chairman, Professor Dr H. C. Rümke, outlined the general plans and the objectives of the Group. These were described in retrospect by Dr J. R. Rees, in his Introduction to *Mental Health in International Perspective* (21), as follows:

> 'The primary task of the Study Group was to make a broad survey of progress being made in the many aspects of the mental health field throughout the world. An attempt was made to cover the spectrum of interest from research and care of the mentally sick at one end, to international relationships at the other. Having made a study of recent experiences, the Study Group aimed to put into perspective some of the major activities that need to be undertaken in various areas of the world during the next decade.'

Readers who are personally concerned with promoting small international group meetings may be interested in the mechanics of programme planning. In its now wide experience of conducting such meetings, WFMH has found that it is very important at the beginning of a conference to allow enough time for the whole programme to be thoroughly discussed. Times of sessions, their duration, free periods, and so on, should be fixed by group decisions. However flexible the plans are in the early stages, we have found it best, once the programme decisions have been made, to adhere to them strictly, so that participants can take on other commitments. Distinguished foreign scientists are always in demand for public engagements in the countries they are visiting, and international conference organizers should make full allowance for this.

The first session was devoted to planning the programme. After considerable discussion of work method, the Study Group adopted a plan of plenary sessions, interspersed with periods when three simultaneous work groups would be discussing the same subject, after which they would report back to the whole group in plenary session for further discussion. The principle in allocating members to work groups was to secure the greatest possible spread by discipline, culture, language, and sex, and at each work-group session a different combination of members was arranged.

The work groups devoted sessions to the following discussion areas:

Clinical matters and prophylaxis
Research
Professional training
Public education in mental health; and mental health implications in other fields of science and professional practice
Mental health and cultural attitudes
Recommendations.

The Study Group met each day for four sessions: 9.0 a.m.–10.30 a.m.; 11.0 a.m.–12.30 p.m.; 2.30 p.m.–4.0 p.m.; and 4.30 p.m.–6.0 p.m. One midweek afternoon was left free in both weeks, and the middle Saturday afternoon and the whole of Sunday were free.

The arrangements made for monitoring and recording are very important ingredients of success. A complete tape recording was made of every session of the Study Group, not because a verbatim report was contemplated, but for reference purposes. However, unless a minute-by-minute note is kept of each speaker, the subject, and the number on the indicator, all that the editor will have to work on at the close will be an amorphous mass of taped material to which there is no guide, and which can be unravelled only by spending as much time listening to it as the original discussion occupied in recording. A good indexing system enables the significant parts of the material to be identified and a permanent record made in any appropriate order. In the present instance, the tapes recorded more than 400,000 words, so that without efficient monitoring the editors would have had an impossible task. In the case of French-speakers, the English interpretation was recorded on the tape for the convenience of the editors, who were working in the English language.

The services of the late Mr Albert Deutsch, a science writer with a life-long experience of interpreting mental health subjects to the more general reader, had been secured to prepare the short monograph or précis to be submitted to the Sixth International Congress on Mental Health in Paris in August 1961. Mr Deutsch's chosen work method was to dictate quietly on a special tape recorder certain comments on the discussion as it took place. These were typed back for his use later. In addition, he signalled to the monitor of the main tape recorder when he wanted any particular passage or series of contributions to be noted for later transcription in full. He had planned in this way to collect enough material to enable him to write his survey of the fortnight's discussion within a few days of its conclusion.

THE ATMOSPHERE OF THE STUDY GROUP

It would be very difficult to give a really adequate description of how the Study Group went about its work, and of its unique atmosphere. There were many positive assets and, perhaps, a minimum of practical difficulties to overcome at the outset. The location was very favourable indeed, there were comfortable quarters, efficient service, good food, and a bar. The gardens and grounds surrounding the house were lovely, and for once in a generation the English June weather lived up to its poetic reputation.

Although the preparatory work had been hurried, there was no lack of background material of high quality, for a great deal of experience of the conduct of small international meetings had gone into its collection. The administrative arrangements were consistently excellent, and the methods of recording and secretarial help were more than adequate. The members of the Study Group are agreed that the whole fortnight went by without a single administrative or domestic difficulty causing inconvenience to any member.

The greatest starting asset of the Study Group was the fact that, by design, all of its members were experienced in international contacts, and in transcultural and cross-disciplinary communication. Most of them had known each other over many years, and those few who were less well personally acquainted with the remainder knew them well by reputation. It was a very important ingredient of later success that all those who accepted the invitation had done so recognizing that the aims of the Study Group had not been explicitly stated, that its projected scope was very wide indeed, and its task manifestly complex.

However sound the planning and however favourable the start and the background circumstances, no interprofessional cross-cultural group could expect to avoid all difficulties and tensions, nor would it be an ultimate advantage to do so. To a certain extent the natural anxiety of this *ad hoc* group, which had come together to tackle a complex job in a period of time that was obviously too short, was countered by the adoption of a clear framework of discussion and a plan of work to which every member agreed. It was also important to resist strong temptations to attempt too much and to give too great a proportion of time to small group discussions. Since the whole group had agreed to the times of sessions, they were adhered to rather strictly, and we are convinced that to continue a discussion after the stated time of closure because it happens to be fruitful at that moment is more likely to create tension than to bring positive results. Members collectively also tended to discourage any group work at other times. There was, of course, plenty of extra work that the participants could do individually, and a large number of important annotations and other comments on the discussion were handed in for inclusion among the material to be considered in the preparation of the extended report.

No group activities were arranged for the free half-days and the middle Sunday. Some members of the Group found the location, four miles from a country town and forty miles from London, rather too remote for a residential meeting of two weeks, and it was difficult for them to accept any outside engagements. As we have remarked, people who are well known internationally are likely to receive a large number of calls on their time from colleagues who wish to take advantage of their presence in the country to arrange a meeting or a lecture. This legitimate aspect of communication in the international field needs to be provided for, as well as the interest of the visitors in the cultural life of the host country.

There was one important source of pressure of which the members of the Group were conscious – the need to produce an agreed statement in time for circulation at the International Congress on Mental Health in Paris two months later. From a purely practical point of view, it is a very big undertaking to write a report of about 20,000 words, check the proofs, and complete the printing and publishing within a period of eight weeks, especially when the period covers the holiday months of July and August. A more ambitious plan, to publish not only the English version but a French translation also, in time for the Paris meeting, proved to be quite impracticable.

The International Preparatory Commission of 1948 had succeeded in publishing a statement that had been agreed by the members in time for distribution at the Third International Congress on Mental Health in London in 1948. But this remarkable feat was achieved at the expense of devoting a great proportion of the latter part of the Commission's time to reaching agreement on the terms of the report. This experience of the 1948 Commission was carefully considered, but in planning the 1961 Group it was decided that it would not be the best use of the time and talents of the members of the Study Group to devote so much attention to reaching agreement on a joint statement. The alternative plan was, as we have stated, to entrust an experienced science journalist with the task of writing an account of the Study Group, for which he would take responsibility and which would be published under his name. In this way it was hoped to relieve the members of the Study Group of the feeling that it was necessary to agree with all that was written in the report, and to free them for more constructive activity. The plan had the major disadvantage that, though the members recognized the sound practical reasons for its adoption, they were not entirely happy about not taking full responsibility for the report which was being written in the Group's name. It was felt that a report written by a professional writer on behalf of a scientific group would have a very different impact from that of an agreed statement of the whole Study Group; it might perhaps be more influential with the educated general public, but almost certainly would be less so in mental health professional circles.

As may be imagined, the sudden death of Mr Deutsch in the early hours of Sunday, 18 July, at the midway point of the meeting, had a profound effect on the atmosphere of the second week of the Study Group. First was the sense of personal grief that every member of the Group experienced at the loss of one whose unique personal qualities and life-long contribution to mental health had made a much-loved figure. Second was a new sense of urgency imparted by the realization that only one week remained in which to work out how the report could be completed. Emergency procedures for the compilation of the first summary report were discussed by the Study Group at the first session of the second week. Two members, who, with the approval of the whole Group, elected to remain anonymous, undertook to continue with the collection of the material in order to write the short report during the three weeks immediately following the Study Group. This had the unfortunate effect of virtually removing these two participants from active discussion, but it was unanimously agreed that much of the impact and usefulness of the whole Study Group would be lost if the preliminary statement were not published as planned.

The task facing these two members was immense, and was made much more difficult by the fact that neither of them had had in mind the collection of material for the short report when they were participating in the first week's discussions. Admittedly, they had access to the notes and excerpts taken by Mr Deutsch, but it is obviously difficult to work with someone else's material, and particularly so when that person had an entirely different orientation, background, and professional objective in undertaking the task.

The other members of the Study Group were very alive to the problems that the two newly appointed editors had been set, and each member undertook to make annotations on the substance and interpretation of the discussions for use, at will, by the editors. However, these annotations, helpful though they were, greatly increased the volume of work, and the editors could get through it only at the price of very many hours of work, day and night. How they completed their task within three weeks of the close of the Study Group is a question only they can answer, if indeed they know themselves. It was a very remarkable feat.

In retrospect it now seems clear that the original decision to appoint a science writer – however well-known to and trusted by the members – to prepare the first report on their behalf had been a source of considerable anxiety to the Study Group as a whole, in spite of the fact that the plan had been freely accepted. At the end of the first week there had been a general awareness of confusion of aim and lack of clarity of purpose. This awareness was suddenly crystallized into anxiety as a result of the emergency that arose.

The Study Group's constructive response to the emergency situation was both a result of and a contributory factor to the increased sense of purposefulness and unity that characterized the atmosphere of the second week, and helped the two editors with their task. In the atmosphere prevailing it was found necessary for the Study Group to spend only a brief time towards the end of the meeting in securing agreement on the main lines of the short report. Final responsibility for the content was left in the hands of the Steering Committee in consultation with the two editors.

It was generally agreed that the feeling of increased purposefulness that the Study Group acquired as a result of these difficulties not only helped those who were writing the reports, but also improved the quality of the Group's work. However, three days later the emotional tension of the Group was again heightened by a further misfortune – Dr Frank Fremont-Smith had to fly home for emergency surgery, from which it was later learnt that he had made an excellent recovery.

In spite of these unforeseen difficulties – the tragic loss of one member and the serious illness of another – the experience of being a member of the Study Group was a memorable one. Indeed, members thought that the 1961 Study Group had perhaps been the most notable event that had yet occurred in the sphere of international mental health work. Certainly, the editors of the current volume, after months of being steeped in the discussion processes of the Group, became convinced that work of very high quality was achieved at Roffey Park in 1961.

'MENTAL HEALTH IN INTERNATIONAL PERSPECTIVE'

The brief volume of some 22,000 words exclusive of the French and Spanish language summaries, which was prepared for distribution at the Paris Congress, contains in clear and succinct form the essence of the work of the International Study Group. It is aimed at a wide range of readership, but the anonymous editors had in mind especially the responsible citizen, without professional qualifications in this field, who may nevertheless have some influence on the mental and social wellbeing of his own community.

THE EXTENDED REPORT

The extended Report in three volumes is intended primarily to give scientific background and authority to the spirit of the Study Group's findings, as distilled in *Mental Health in International Perspective*. Compilation has been the responsibility of Dr Kenneth Soddy, Director of the Study Group project and Secretary to the Scientific Committee of WFMH, and of Dr Robert H. Ahrenfeldt, Consultant to the Study Group project, with the assistance of Miss Mary C. Kidson, Technical Assistant to the Scientific Division, WFMH, and Administrator of the Study Group project. During the second week of the Study Group, part of a session was devoted to consideration of the main structure, in principle, of the extended Report, but beyond this no work was done on the Report during the meeting by the Study Group itself.

The preparation of this Report has been a very complex task.

The raw materials included the following sources: tape recordings of all the plenary discussions, monitored at the time of recording and later indexed; tape recordings of the group discussions, which were less useful because not monitored and so to some extent duplicated in later plenary sessions; précis writers' reports of the plenary sessions; working papers contributed by participants; annotations produced during the meeting; and the background material that had been circulated beforehand.

The editorial process included three main tasks: first, the completion of the bibliography, the groundwork for which had already been done by Dr Ahrenfeldt during the course of the preliminary preparations; second, the rearrangement of the taped material according to the main structure of the Report decided on by the Study Group; and third, the further ordering of the material according to its own structure and dynamics as they developed.

The précis writers' reports were a very valuable aid in the rearrangement process and enabled the editors quickly to discover where material could be found on the tapes. The précis were rapidly scanned and the paragraphs on each definable topic were cut out and allocated to the appropriate section, care being taken to put an identity mark on each cutting. By the appropriate ordering of these fragments, which were then connected with relevant parts of working papers, it was possible to build up the general structure of each chapter. The subject-matter was then written in, with the précis as a guide, but with reference to the tapes for the substance, which was paraphrased or quoted according to circumstances.

The object of this procedure was to ensure that nothing would be included in the Report that had not been aired and discussed by the Study Group itself, except for certain quotations that have been made *in extenso* from documents that were available and referred to by members of the Study Group.

A draft of each chapter was circulated to members of the Study Group in order to obtain comments and suggestions for incorporation into a second draft. This long and complex process has, no doubt, delayed publication by many months, but as a result it has become possible to issue the extended Report with the authority of the Study Group. Such authority does not imply that every member of the Study Group agrees with every word that has been written, but it is the conviction of the editors that nothing has been included to which any member of the Group has made known an objection, except in the case of those passages which have been ascribed to an individual or a minority view. The editors believe that members of the Study Group are fully in accord with the great mass of material in these volumes, and, in particular, with the spirit and attitudes expressed.

3
Summary of Recommendations

The Study Group discussed a number of recommendations submitted by individual members, with the intention, originally, of preparing agreed statements which it was hoped might carry some weight with administrators and others working in the field of mental health and human welfare. We have remarked above on the impact made by the recommendations of the 1948 International Preparatory Commission. It was agreed, however, that the climate of work in the mental health field had changed considerably and that, for example, in comparison with 1948 there was now far more organized activity, especially international and intercultural cooperation. Whereas in 1948 a series of recommendations had had the effect of stimulating thought and action, a similar list of recommendations made in 1961 could hardly prove as fruitful.

After considerable discussion, the consensus of opinion in the 1961 Study Group was that while some useful purpose might be served by bringing to the notice of organizations and individuals certain important fields of work that would repay attention, it was not the role of the WFMH Study Group to suggest to other organizations what ought to be done. Therefore the Study Group restricted itself to commenting on work that needed doing, and wished to make it clear that if any definite recommendations were implied in its observations, they would be directed specifically to the World Federation for Mental Health.

COLLABORATION IN TRANSNATIONAL ACTIVITIES

The Study Group noted many examples of successful collaboration between the various United Nations agencies, their regional offices, and voluntary agencies in the mental health field. The hope was expressed that such collaboration could be both expanded and intensified, and it was remarked that WFMH would welcome an expansion of the specific mental health activities of the UN agencies. There has been a marked tendency recently for more attention to be paid to mental health needs, and, more designedly, for mental health projects to be included in the technical assistance programmes of UN and the similar operations of other agencies. It is greatly to be hoped that there will be still further developments along these lines. An outstanding example has been the mental health services for refugees provided by UN agencies.

Among the recommendations in *Mental Health and World Citizenship* (12) is the establishment of assessment agencies for international technical aid projects. The 1961 Study Group endorsed the view of the 1948 Commission in this respect, and was impressed by the importance of including arrangements for continuous operational assessment as an integral part of all such programmes.

Of no less importance is the improvement of methods of selection of personnel to go abroad on technical aid and other missions involving exacting responsibilities in cultures other than their own and in unfamiliar conditions. In no field is this more important than in that of international relations.

The Study Group was of the opinion that there had been insufficient exchange of plans and general information among the agencies undertaking mental health projects transnationally, and drew attention to the importance of inter-agency discussions at national and international levels in all fields of activity related to mental health. The promotion of expert groups or symposia appears to be the best way of improving communication between the workers in these fields. Three main priorities are recommended:

(a) the definition of those fields of activity in which there is at the present time sufficient knowledge and skill for taking appropriate action, and the drawing up of plans that can be put into operation at once;

(b) the definition of those areas where present knowledge and skill, though admittedly incomplete, appear to be the best available, and the encouragement of action at the present time, based on existing experience but in the full recognition of the limitations of knowledge;

(c) the definition of those areas in which it is clear that any immediate action would be premature, given the present state of knowledge.

TRANSNATIONAL RESEARCH PROJECTS

At the international level, mental health research shows little or no evidence of pattern in organization, and the Study Group was convinced that many opportunities for valuable new work are not being taken at present. This situation is drawn to the attention of WFMH with the remark that it is timely, or perhaps more than timely, to set about the establishment of one or more international research institutes in order to encourage and sponsor projects as occasions for effective action arise. The functions of these research institutes would be to plan transnational research projects in collaboration with local centres in groups of countries; to make available the services of key research personnel around whom the teams could be collected; to act as a channel, through which local finance could be made available for projects; and, perhaps most important, to take part in the training of local workers and to act as consultants in local planning and supervision. Valuable contributions could be made by arranging meetings of scientists at the international level as a means of sponsoring the exchange of information, by organizing training fellowships, and by providing an expert service on the design and execution of research projects requiring transnational operation.

As part of their information service, the institutes might establish international registers of research on mental health. This could be part of a clearing-house function for research information, but the Study Group was not convinced of the essential usefulness of an exchange of information service or clearing house on its own, in isolation and not as part of a programme of planning, action, and training in research; especially if more than one culture is to be covered. At the very least, the personnel of such an information exchange should themselves possess the necessary training and experience to enable them to provide, as a service, guides for operational research in various fields of work, including the early exploration of problems in the establishment of mental health services where none has existed previously. At best, the information exchange should earn and enjoy the prestige that attaches to an institution that has a reputation for making original contributions to scientific knowledge.

NATIONAL MENTAL HEALTH ORGANIZATIONS

The Study Group reaffirmed and again drew the attention of WFMH to the recommendation of the 1948 International Preparatory Commission that national mental health bodies be established in every country for service, education, and research. The hope was expressed that UN agencies would do all that is in their power to help such activities to develop.

It was felt that WFMH is well placed to take leading action in the training of personnel to serve as mental health association executives or leaders, and to foster or undertake studies of the roles of mental health professional people in the various social institutions that significantly affect human behaviour. Such essential training activities could be made more effective as a result of further studies of the basic material from various fields, including psychology, sociology, and biology, that is suitable for inclusion in the training of people who are working in the human sciences.

INTERNATIONAL CONFERENCES

The Study Group considered that a very valuable contribution had been made to contemporary mental health action by the organization of small expert conferences on subjects of particular relevance to the current situation, and deplored an apparent diminution in such fruitful activities during the past two or three years. In the wide field of action of mental health there are numerous subjects that would well repay treatment in like manner. Given the existing state of development of many countries, the Study Group felt that the following areas of work were of especial importance at that time:

(a) The question of work satisfaction in an increasingly automated society; the effect on family life of changes in economic circumstances resulting from a shift from a subsistence economy to an industrial economy, from craft employment to mass production; automation and the role of the unskilled worker; and the problems of increasing leisure and increasing spending power. Not only are these problems of particular interest to mental health associations but they also closely concern UNESCO and the UN Social Commission. It would, for example, be valuable to prepare a handbook on mental health principles in these areas, for the use of industrial personnel workers.

(b) Problems in relation to increased expectation of life, including the prolongation of life of handicapped people. This complex area of social activity includes the widening of the life of handicapped people, and their increased potential in productive activity with modern methods of rehabilitation and automation; the mental health aspects of rigid retirement laws or regulations that may be out of date in modern society; and the effect on society as a whole, and on family life and balance, of the increasing proportion of elderly people.

The Study Group recommended the convening of an expert meeting which might possibly lead up to an annual meeting of WFMH devoted to problems arising out of the current increased intimacy of contact and complexity of relationships among people of different race, culture, etc.; and also concerned with the study of the genesis of antagonisms leading to group conflict, prejudice, and discriminatory attitudes, and with relevant prophylactic action.

MENTAL HEALTH SUBJECTS FOR FURTHER STUDY

The Study Group considered a number of significant areas in which, in its opinion, further research is required before definitive programmes of action can be drawn up. This does not imply that no activity should be undertaken in any of the following spheres. On the contrary, wherever a contribution can be usefully made, however incompletely, it is important to attempt it, just as it is important not to go to the other extreme and cease further investigation into a subject because by common consent it has been added to the area of current practical activity. Areas of concern which are particularly relevant for further study at the present time are:

(a) *Theoretical Concepts of Change*

After some discussion of the major question of the world-wide phenomenon of change in social and individual life, the Study Group was impressed by the serious lack of precise knowledge in this area, and recommended that theoretical concepts concerning change and the adjustment of the individual should be submitted to radical multidisciplinary study. The Study Group recommended further consideration of the hypothesis that change may be effected in the individual not so much by a process of adjustment to changing circumstances as by a process of absorption and growth in such a way that a new stream of culture is incorporated into the structure of the personality which, however, maintains its essential continuity. By this approach there might be developed a concept of self-realization through change instead of a concept of change by adaptation and alteration.

The concept of absorption of change implies a different notion of identity-formation – one that would enable a greater flexibility of personality development. The Study Group made the further recommendation that the new concept of absorption of change might be applicable by analogy to intergroup relationships: thus when two different communities are brought into close contact with each other, instead of each community being compelled to adapt its behaviour to the changed conditions, each may come to accept the presence of the other party as part of its own total identity. A new theoretical concept of nationhood is put forward for urgent consideration – that a nation does not attain the full stature of its identity until it has incorporated in its system of relationships the presence of other nations. Thus, the total identity of each nation would be dependent on the full and independent coexistence of others.

One practical application of the foregoing is to consider whether the concept of absorption of change may invalidate the common assumption that rapid cultural change necessarily and automatically constitutes a stress situation. The theoretical proposition is advanced that a community may be able to pass rapidly from a primitive state of organization to one of a complex modern society without undue stress, provided that transitional periods and areas of partial change in the community do not occur, in which living habits develop that are indicative of social malaise, e.g. new slum areas in industrial cities. This theoretical concept is of such potential significance that its detailed study is urgent.

(b) *Studies of Intergroup Relations in Society*

The Study Group recommended that intensive examination be given to the question of the relationship between conflict situations and destructive aggression, in order to test the hypothesis that it may be the conflict situations that release aggressive impulses otherwise under control rather than the reverse process in which the conflict arises out of inherent aggressiveness. This hypothesis, if proved, might make it possible to remove the danger of war, by enabling social patterns to be devised that would obviate conflict situations; an approach that might be more hopeful than concentration on the prevention or control of destructive aggression.

It is recommended that further comparative studies be undertaken of adolescents in several societies, with the aim of throwing light upon intergroup relationships and communication. Among the many aspects of this subject may be noted: (i) certain problems of behaviour that occur in societies where the adolescent peer group appears to be relatively cut off from the main cultural influences in the society; (ii) the stress that derives in some modern societies from the extension of the period of compulsory education beyond adolescence into young adulthood, and may give rise to acute behaviour problems; (iii) behaviour problems that are associated with tendencies in the opposite direction in other societies – tendencies that demand adult behaviour of adolescents prematurely.

(c) *Prevention*

It appeared to the Study Group that virtually no field of prevention had been adequately opened up by scientific investigation. The following areas of study are selected as being of particular relevance to modern conditions, and are offered as examples of work that needs to be done.

There has been a striking lack of attention given to the question of the various conditions that permit optimum mental health of individuals in their existing circumstances. This subject needs to be tackled on a wide basis of study and action, of which the latter includes the promotion of knowledge of mental health principles among those with responsibilities in the community.

The problem of the early recognition of behaviour that is affected by stress to which the individual cannot adapt, and also by incipient mental disorder or borderline deficiency, was discussed at length in the Study Group. It was agreed that efforts in the direction of earlier recognition of disorders through refinement of diagnostic techniques and rationalization of psychiatric nomenclature deserved all support. The Group was particularly interested in the incorporation of interdisciplinary procedures and the involvement of social institutions in the attempt to discern trouble at an earlier stage. It was recommended to WFMH that it would be useful to hold an annual meeting on this subject, especially if the meeting were to be preceded by a coordinated study in a number of countries; and in this connexion the Study Group drew attention to the valuable work of WHO and other interested bodies in epidemiological studies of mental disorders. Work in this field includes long-range follow-up studies, and researches in the basic sciences in order to develop more precise diagnostic techniques. The clinical trial and assessment of new therapeutic techniques under strict conditions also have a valuable potential contribution to make to prevention.

To three specific areas of study in the field of prevention the Study Group gave high priority:

(i) the determination of 'indicators' of imminent social or individual breakdown relating to a given community;
(ii) the 'case-finding' training of professional people, and the 'case-recognition' education of the public;
(iii) the identification of those people in the community who are vulnerable under conditions of social change, and the more precise examination of the agents to which they are susceptible.

The very considerable increase in many countries in admissions to mental hospitals and the rapid turnover of patients have given rise to problems that need further study, e.g. the possible exacerbation of social maladjustment or prolongation of inadequacy as the result of the discharge from hospital of psychotic patients in a very early stage of recovery. Further, in places where mental hospitals pursue an active policy of treatment and discharge, the problem of the social deterioration of the chronic hospital patient may become relatively more important. Comparatively little is known about the effects of long hospitalization.

In those countries or areas in which there have been no facilities for psychiatric therapy, but in which through the opening up of communication and contact with other cultures a demand for the introduction of psychiatric services is arising, there may be calls for immediate action in respect of persons who are newly recognized to be suffering from serious psychiatric disorder. The Study Group recommended that close attention be given to the possibility of providing simple sheltering agencies for those who, in default of full psychiatric treatment, would benefit from kindly but informed nursing care for their maladies. However, such action would be justified only when it was planned as the first step in the introduction of adequate psychiatric services. It should be regarded as a device to cover a period in which an awakening social conscience demands action, at a time when the facilities for a full therapeutic programme are not available.

There are currently unique opportunities, of which full advantage should be taken, to study certain spontaneously occurring phenomena in a number of cultures, especially the emergence of new social institutions in rapidly developing and changing countries.

One emerging social institution of profound contemporary significance is that of universal literacy through the rapid growth of educational systems throughout the world, in which connexion the particular point for study would be the effects on society of the introduction of compulsory full-time school attendance for children. As each decade passes there will be fewer and fewer opportunities for the analysis of this radical social innovation. The Study Group drew attention to the need for more scientifically planned research concerning the training of teachers, and particularly of educational administrators and those promoting educational programmes. It is essential, from the mental health point of view, to secure congruence between educational and other social development, e.g. employment opportunities.

Wherever education is expanding, it is very important to recognize the increasing share of responsibility for the mental health of future generations that is being carried by teachers and school administrators, because more children are spending longer periods of time in school. The main questions for study are: how the professional training of teachers may be improved in respect of their capacity to use educational methods to promote personality development among the children through the learning process; and how the teachers' ability to recognize signs of maladjustment and difficulty among children may be increased. Recognition is not enough in this case, for, in addition, teachers need to be well informed about the community resources upon which they may call for assistance once a problem is known to exist, and the resources themselves need to be adequate to the demands that will be made on them.

The last, but not the least important, of the recommendations for study and action made by the 1961 Study Group was in support of far more research than has yet been undertaken into the human factors involved in the possibility of accident in connexion with nuclear armaments. The Study Group considered that among these factors may be included: the psychological effects of isolation on the individuals concerned; their unique position in society through the possession of knowledge and skill, with immense potentiality for destruction; and the acute dangers attending the attainment of positions of responsibility and power in this connexion by people with paranoid personality tendencies.

costs and the resources themselves, and to the safeguards as to the manner that will be made of them.

[illegible]

PART TWO

Mental Health Trends in a Changing World

4
World Citizenship and a New Concept of Nationhood

It would be a mammoth undertaking to review comprehensively the trends reflected in the mental health literature published since the report of the International Preparatory Commission of 1948. Far from being a comprehensive review, the preparatory work done for the International Study Group of 1961 represents no more than a general look at some of the more easily recognized trends.

The first impression gained from a survey of the literature is that, with certain notable exceptions, in most of the areas little significant new work is to be found. By far the greater part of the original studies are concerned with clinical problems and other research of a restricted, technical nature. The literature on important national, international, and cross-cultural aspects of mental health consists mainly of somewhat generalized views and considerations, some of which have been the subject of interprofessional discussion, but more usually in a single or limited cultural setting.

Much of the leadership in international work in mental health since the end of World War II has been given by two international organizations: WFMH (1948), and WHO (Mental Health Section, 1949); with the cooperation, on a number of occasions, of other United Nations agencies (UNESCO, ILO, etc.), and of various national, as well as international (non-governmental) organizations (3, 4, 36).

There is no lack of interest in the transnational aspects of mental health work. On the contrary, there is evidence of a widespread willingness both to share new advances and to learn from the experience of others. But while much of the literature that we have looked at displays a perhaps not wholly justified confidence in the value of transcultural communication in this field, several authors have warned about the complexity of these matters, and against any facile assumption of 'universally' applicable plans, generalizations, or alleged solutions in the field of practical mental health work. It was in response to a growing recognition that to be mentally healthy may have quite different meanings for different people and cultures that the Scientific Committee of WFMH devoted its second cross-cultural study, *Mental Health and Value Systems* (41), to making an inquiry into the compatibility of contemporary mental health concepts with various religions and ideologies.

An example of the practical application of this recognition can be found in the words of an anthropologist member of the Study Group:

> 'Particular caution is necessary when, by virtue of the geographical and economic situation, health personnel from several different cultures are gathered together under the heading of "South East Asia" or "The Caribbean". Such areas do have much in common, but the finer differences in family structure, in ethos, in world view, tend to be obscured in overall statements. . . . There is a danger that the preservation of a careful and explicit respect for differences in cultures may give rise to stereotypes about East and West – stereotypes which have been originated in Western, urban, industrialized, or middle-class cultural attitudes and are then projected upon, and eventually incorporated by, those members of the new nations who are oriented towards modern industrialized societies.'

It is too early to view and assess in truly historical perspective the mental health problems and activities of the last decade. Indeed, it is only relatively recently that we have had comprehensive accounts and evaluations of the *entire* range of historical evolution of science and medicine (by Sarton, Sigerist, Singer, Garrison, Castiglioni, *et al.*), and of psychiatry in the past few centuries (e.g. in the works of Semelaigne, Laignel-Lavastine,

Vinchon, and Zilboorg). Apart from a few instances (comparable, say, with the discovery of sulphonamides and antibiotics in our own lifetime), we cannot yet say what will in due course be shown to have been significant landmarks in the advance of the mental health sciences; this is as dynamic and evolutionary a process as human history itself.

Dr E. E. Krapf observed:

> 'Mental health work necessarily requires a multidisciplinary effort in which all branches of the sciences of man . . . should be equal partners. Perhaps one of the greatest benefits of the international approach to mental health matters is that it can show the psychiatrist the limitations of his field and teach him a measure of humility' (3).

There may, perhaps, be no better dedication of our efforts in the field of mental health than that inscribed in one of the later works (10) of the eminent French psychiatrist, René Semelaigne – to the younger generation:

> *. . . et le meilleur souhait qu'il me soit possible de leur adresser est de savoir unir l'effort de l'heure présente, l'espoir des jours futurs, au culte du passé.* ('. . . and the best wish I can possibly make for them is that they may know how to unite their effort at the present time, and their hope for the days to come, with a reverence for the past.')

The 1961 Study Group took as its starting point the statement issued by its predecessor, the International Preparatory Commission of 1948, on *Mental Health and World Citizenship* (12). In the 1948 document we read, 'Perhaps what we are stating represents a vision rather than a rigid scientific demonstration'. This, it was thought, could still be regarded as the main aim of the 1961 Study Group, but it would be necessary to adopt an entirely new approach. The background to the earlier statement had been the second world war, and those who attended the 1948 meeting were still preoccupied with the tremendous mental health problems of war's immediate aftermath. Much has happened since that era.

It was considered that the 1948 report, written in the shadow of war, perhaps left an impression that its writers thought that unless world citizenship was achieved and international human relations improved there was a great risk of total extermination. In 1961 it was generally agreed that, owing to the enormous developments in nuclear destructive power and in methods of chemical and biological warfare, the risk of total annihilation that faced the world was considerably greater than in 1948. Yet we feel that it is our job to point to the altered conditions, rather than to prophesy doom because of a feared failure in human relations. Not only have the possibilities of total destruction increased, but also, as a result of improved means of communication, the whole world is living at much closer range than was the case even in 1948; and this, in turn, necessarily involves a greater interdependence, a greater sharing of fortune, both good and evil. Thus, to an increasing degree, the whole world must share in the destruction of part of it. This makes us all, in a real sense and to some extent, the guardians of the safety of all other people.

Our duty, therefore, is to do our best to alert the world to a new situation that has come into existence with the development of nuclear weapons and other methods of destruction, and to dangers that appear to have become aggravated since that time.

WORLD CITIZENSHIP

In making suggestions as to how steps could be taken towards the attainment of a higher standard of world citizenship and the improvement of the quality of effort being made on behalf of mental health the world over, *Mental Health and World Citizenship* has not been ineffective. It may be claimed that every one of the many practical recommendations included in the report has been implemented, in part or in whole, somewhere in the world. But in spite of its eminently practical aim and effect and the brilliance of its summary of the world situation, the report has had some adverse as well as beneficial effects. Many people in the mental health field have been repelled rather than attracted by the attitude expressed in the 1948 document. These issues will be discussed more fully below and in Volume II. The Study Group, in 1961, was far more concerned to contribute towards understanding by elucidation of the psychodynamic forces involved. For example, in discussing problems of prejudice, discrimination, and segregation, it was our concern to work out the underlying psychodynamic mechanisms and draw attention to these, rather than to recommend what people should do in particular circumstances.

Mental Health and World Citizenship needs reinterpretation in many important respects, one of these being the degree to which the goals and values of the individual and the particular community are becoming progressively influenced by those of other people and communities. In the 1948 statement it was pointed out that the adequacy of the concept of world citizenship that the individual may have depends upon the quality of his own citizenship. It appeared to the 1961 Study Group that this view is still valid and that our function today is to do what we can to help people, nationally or locally, to work out their own values for themselves. One practical way of doing this is the promotion of a sense of citizenship in a community by spreading knowledge of other people, their achievements and their problems. It is to be hoped that knowledge of what is happening in other parts of the world will help some people to avoid difficulties and mistakes into which others have fallen, and to undertake new work that otherwise would not be initiated. This concept of the function of mental health goes beyond the question of mental illness or, as one member of the Group phrased it, 'social or economic engineering'.

The notion of world citizenship propounded in the 1948 statement seems to have implied the subordination of individual national or regional citizenship to the interests of the whole world, which concept necessarily involves the resolution of conflicting ideas of independence and sovereignty on the one hand, and mutual support and interdependence on the other.

Our present concern is with the dynamics of extension of the sense of citizenship from the personal loyalties of the individual to family, clan, and nation, to the wider field of humanity. To illustrate only one of many sets of conflicting attitudes in this field: some people see the extreme position of individual freedom and independence as being attainable only at the expense of a sense of collective responsibility. Others, on the contrary, believe that the maximum degree of freedom and independence can be obtained only by the exercise of a high degree of personal responsibility which regards the rights and needs of others equally with those of the individual.

The Study Group, however much it might be interested in some of these philosophical ideas, sought not to go beyond making statements that were within its scientific competence. For example, instead of making an idealistic statement about world citizenship, the 1961 Group considered it more proper to restrict itself to the remark that ideas of national independence, sovereignty, and self-interest that were perfectly tenable two hundred years ago might spell disaster, at least to somebody, if pursued now, because of the changed conditions in which humanity is living. This is not a statement of ideals or philosophy but, rather, a technically justified statement based on objective observation of living conditions in the world today. However, it is an important duty, having made this remark, to attempt, in addition, to contribute more constructively to the resolution of the problems involved.

It appeared to the Study Group that there is no scientific evidence that it is possible for the concept of citizenship to spread outwards by the extension of personal relations to the world community. It may be necessary, rather, to aim at building up the sense of nationhood in such a way that the national integrity of other nations becomes an important factor in the individual's own nationhood. This is the analogy in the international sphere of the notion of the empathic individual as expressed by the seventeenth-century English philosopher and poet, John Donne: 'Every man's death diminishes me.' Owing to the interdependence of nations in the world today, destruction of or severe damage suffered by one nation, whether friendly, temporarily hostile, or traditionally inimical, harms all other nations in contact; and the network of contact in the modern world is very widespread.

An educationalist pointed out that in the 1948 report (p. 25) the idea of the world citizen is meant to convey the notion of a common humanity. He said:

> 'Common humanity can be expressed and experienced only through diversity, and every diversity must have an identity; and therefore the preservation of identities, which has been referred to, is fundamental to the whole idea of human association. The infant and the mother are concerned to preserve the identity of each other in order that they may preserve their own, and things are reciprocally related in that way. Family life is possible because each is concerned to preserve his own identity by preserving the identity of the others. They are bound up together. This is what we mean by interdependence. In the same way, to have a "good" society the individual has to be concerned about preserving the identity of his neighbour; we can envisage a "good" world only in terms of groups being concerned to preserve each other's identity. The welfare of the whole cannot be considered apart from the welfare of the separate parts.'

There has been no word in common use to express the idea of 'good' national behaviour, though recently the term 'nationhood' has been introduced in this context. Throughout the twentieth century the word 'nationalism' has been acquiring an increasingly pejorative meaning. It would be just to remark that nationalism has come to be regarded as an evil force when applied to the patriotic activities of other national groups felt to be hostile to the observer; but that similar antagonistic activities of one's own are felt to be morally admissible and are not termed nationalistic.

Our concern is with the possibilities of developing a new kind of nationhood, which is not so much an allegiance to the world community as a system of national identity formation by which each individual member of each nation has some kind of personal stake in the existence and wellbeing of all other nations.

The importance to the future of the world of a new outlook on national feeling has been greatly increased during the last half-century by the vast improvement in communications and greatly increased rapidity of travel. The attitudes of members of different subcultural groups towards each other, today, matter very considerably. Up to now, although attitudes of prejudice and discrimination against other cultural groups, and especially against minorities, have followed certain well-recognized and long-established forms, the amount of harm that they have done has been limited and localized because, for the great mass of people in most countries, foreign groups have not impinged closely on the individual. Today almost everybody all over the world is liable to be brought into close contact with representatives of other societies and groups, so that the potential for harm of discriminatory attitudes is almost limitless.

It was an impression of members of the Study Group that discriminatory attitudes are becoming more widespread. For example, it is self-evident that an increased public consciousness about these matters must exist in those countries where, on the one hand, frankly discriminatory legislation is being enacted or, on the other hand, campaigns to reduce discriminatory legislation and social segregation practices are being conducted in public.

The Study Group was of the opinion that this increase of social consciousness about discrimination and the like is among the most important of the social factors affecting mental health activities today as they cross cultural frontiers. This subject will be referred to again below (p. 104) and discussed more fully in Volume II. Here we shall limit ourselves to the remark that discriminatory attitudes are quite evidently not the prerogative of any one group, although they appear to have had a longer history and their contingent activities a greater degree of organization among certain groups than among others. These phenomena are sometimes referred to as 'racialism' or, as we prefer, 'racism', which term is usually used imprecisely, in the sense of an attitude that derogates other groups on the ground of colour or ethnic origin. There is nothing new, of course, in the rise of such attitudes, but it appears that improved communications have made them more widely dispersed.

Of perhaps more recent origin has been the rise of what is sometimes referred to as 'racialism (or racism) in reverse', though this is equally an imprecise term. This phenomenon has to do with the attitudes towards their persecutors that may be engendered in a group that has been discriminated against, and/or may, in some instances, have been a factor in the genesis of persecutory attitudes in the first place. It is a logical conclusion that discriminatory attitudes represent a mental health problem no less when they are held by black people in respect of white than when they are held by white people in respect of black, or by a religious minority in respect of the majority, and vice versa. Such reverse attitudes to race discrimination have had, on the whole, mainly negative results, at least as far as international cooperation for human welfare is concerned. But there is a more positive aspect, today, in the new sense of participation in the United Nations and in other international councils that is now developing among many peoples that have previously been excluded. This new feeling is contributing something valuable to the sense of identity of those groups whose social situation until recently has been disadvantageous.

It may be argued that in discussing reverse attitudes to race discrimination it is necessary to make a sharp distinction between the racism displayed by previously oppressed peoples—who may themselves be on the way to becoming oppressors—and the sense of pride of belonging to a well-established group. The African races, including those now in the Caribbean, have suffered in consequence of their colour, and virtually all of them are currently reacting, some by a nationalism and racism that may derive in varying proportions from the best and the worst motivations, but others by a search for what is most valuable in their own ethnic group, yet without feeling impelled into conflict with others. This latter attitude is made possible by accepting and bringing to realization the potentialities of one's own particular racial inheritance.

It may be concluded that the 1948 statement implied that world citizenship was a necessary condition for human survival, but that this did not exclude the individual's having loyalty to other entities. The 1961 Study Group endorsed this attitude, with the additional emphasis introduced above that the quality of the individual's concept of world citizenship is to some extent dependent on the quality of his more local loyalties. In spite of the common belief that local and world loyalty must necessarily conflict, there are encouraging signs that to accept and to bring to full realization the individual country's or person's inheritance are more widely becoming regarded as necessary steps towards a world citizenship that is more securely based.

ATTITUDES TO AGGRESSION, DESTRUCTION, AND WAR

The Study Group discussed the suggestion introduced by one of its members that aggression and destructiveness have been linked together in psychological thinking more closely than the facts justify. It was agreed that a clear distinction should be made between aggression and destructiveness, while recognizing that in some circumstances they will combine and augment each other. Although it is obviously true that aggressive impulses are capable of serving those who want war, it by no means follows that, because human beings have inherent aggressive impulses, war is inevitable, though statements of this order are commonly made.

We shall be returning to a fuller discussion of this question in Volume II, and our intention here is only to outline the problem. That destructiveness and aggressiveness in behaviour can vary widely over periods within a single community may be illustrated by the example of India, where the prevailing philosophy of non-violence has been so strongly influential for many centuries that the functions of aggressive behaviour and violence have become canalized into certain martial classes, and the great bulk of the population has lived remarkably pacifically. However, during the partition of India and Pakistan it has been estimated that no fewer than 300,000 people lost their lives through violence, and it is known that a high proportion of these killings were at the hands of essentially pacifically-minded Hindus. Similarly, the island of Bali, for centuries one of the most pacific places in the world, was the scene of remarkably bloodthirsty uprisings against the Dutch rule early in this century, and against the Japanese in 1942. It appears that people with a strictly passive tradition tend on occasion to behave more violently and more destructively than those who have enjoyed a certain legitimization by society of their aggressive and destructive impulses as a normal part of life.

It is clear that the term 'aggression', in its modern usage, needs careful redefinition. At the Third International Congress on Mental Health in 1948, in a series of reports by Frederick Allen, Lauretta Bender, and others, a common view was taken that, as far as emotional relationships are concerned, aggression is a neutral quality, in which a hostile element is not necessarily present.

It is a fact that no school of psychology has been able to demonstrate conclusively that a hostile element in aggression is either universal or inevitable. This appears to have been Freud's own position, in that he spoke of the possibility of eliminating war, while at the same time he held the view that, in principle, the various forms of aggression must necessarily demonstrate their presence. Attempts by psychologists to relate the genesis of war to experience of frustration in early childhood, to unconscious motivation, and to the expression of aggression later in life, have not been convincing. The very fact that some form of compulsion is necessary in order to get boys to fight in any national war is suggestive evidence against an assumption that war represents an outpouring of a natural aggression which must inevitably find expression in that particular manner. Although no one would deny that there are many unsolved problems of control and direction of natural aggression, both individual and group, this does not imply that there is an inevitable or even a direct link between man's aggressive impulses and the phenomenon of warfare.

This vital question is all the more important now that for the first time in history the annihilation of mankind is being conceived as a practical possibility. Although forebodings of world disaster can currently be heard on all sides, it should be remembered that prophecies of the devastation of the human race have followed the discovery of many new types of destructive weapon when they have first been introduced. At the same time, we must not blind our eyes to the immense destructive capacity of nuclear weapons, the long-term (including genetic) effects of widespread radio-activity, and the effect on human life and food production of modern methods of chemical and biological warfare. It would be a totally nihilistic attitude to hold that human aggression leads inevitably to destructiveness and warfare, at a time when human beings, living in close contact with each other everywhere, are equipped with such means of mutual ruin. Therefore it is profoundly important to learn more about the natural history of individual aggressiveness before coming to any such conclusion.

5
Changing Attitudes

The current possibilities both for unprecedented good and for irretrievable ill in the world situation make questions of attitudes, and the changing of attitudes, to peace and war, to working for the good or for the destruction of humanity, of paramount importance.

In discussing changes of attitude, the Study Group started with two premises: that, in general, such changes are the result of many factors; and that it is not a primary mental health objective to arrive at a group consensus, however important it may be to secure changes in attitude. The first problem is how to define adequate criteria of change. As an illustration, an educationalist remarked that in Great Britain, thirty years ago, community interest in children was mainly focused on the child's development and on problems that might arise in the course of growing up, whereas interest has now shifted to the correlated sphere of how adults are to handle the problems with which they are faced in the upbringing of children. This shift has led also to concern about the mental health of parents and teachers. It might be very difficult to demonstrate by any strict criteria that such an attitude change has occurred, yet there are few people working in the field who would have doubts about it. The essence of this example of change is an appreciation of the adults' own problems related to their responsibility for children, and of the interdependence of these concerns. Pointers to the change that are demonstrable to some extent are: a greatly increased interest in the teaching of personality development to students of education; greater understanding of the inherent and intrinsic relationship of development to all aspects of learning (618); and an increase in conscious concern with student mental health.

A child psychiatrist agreed with the impression that there had been an attitude change, which in a number of countries had been little short of revolutionary, among people concerned with child life in the last thirty years. There seem to have been converging movements from child welfare, child guidance, and the education of handicapped children, at the same time as an alerting of public consciousness to mental health work. Mental health organizations have been involved only recently in these affairs – as catalysts rather than originators. For example, the World Federation for Mental Health and the World Health Organization together can justly claim to have exerted some catalytic effect, through the Chichester Seminar of 1952 on Mental Health and Infant Development (510), and the Baguio Seminar of 1958 on Mental Health and Family Life in Asia (434). One indication of a more enlightened cooperative attitude was that, of the governments invited to participate in the seminars, all, without exception, nominated their key people in public health, psychiatry, nursing, child welfare, and education to attend, with the avowed object of later promoting attitude changes in their own countries. Not the least significant outcome has been a network of communication across the world of people who have found a new orientation and a common interest in their widely separate responsibilities.

There are indications, too, of a wide range of change in the attitudes in many countries towards both private and corporate responsibility, particularly in such matters as the provision of social services and the handling of crime. Though it is often difficult for the ordinary citizen to get a balanced view on crime, particularly where violence and destruction are involved, the way in which these matters are reported in the world's press suggests an increasing realization that criminal behaviour tends to come and go in waves which cross national boundaries and involve whole regions, if not most of the world. About 1961 a wave of violent crime affected many countries, and in some of them evidence has been found to relate this 'epidemic' to the wartime experiences of children. Yet efforts to follow up this and other promising leads are almost everywhere hampered by the anxiety of legislators, and those who form public opinion, to name a cause and apply a remedy, however stereotyped. This is one of the many examples of the complexity of the question of changing attitudes, which will be discussed more fully in Volume III.

POPULAR ATTITUDES TO PSYCHIATRIC DIFFICULTIES AND THEIR TREATMENT

Attitudes in the community towards psychiatry, mental disorder, and deviant behaviour in general have not been adequately studied and analysed, even in the more developed countries; still less have popular reactions to the onslaught of empirically based propaganda on mental health been accurately evaluated.

It now appears likely that, in the course of social evolution and as a result of generally available education, popular attitudes and prejudices in this field have been appreciably modified among relatively large sections of the people, at least in countries of Western Europe, North America, and other culturally related countries; but such changes have been, and are, necessarily a slow process.

Thus, in the United Kingdom in 1957 the Royal Commission (404) noted:

> 'There is clearly a strong feeling among the general public . . . that many patients who are now certified could be given the treatment and care they need without certification. . . . While there has been a general increase in public sympathy towards mentally ill patients and a wider understanding of the fact that mental illnesses are . . . usually susceptible to treatment . . . certification seems to have attracted to itself the prejudice and misunderstanding which at one time surrounded the whole idea of mental disorder. It is often thought to imply life-long mental instability, or to carry a social stigma both for the patient and for his family which may persist even after the patient leaves hospital, and to cast doubts on his mental or even on his moral reliability throughout his life, and perhaps on the mental stability of his children and other near relatives.'

On the other hand, in the United States, the Joint Commission on Mental Illness and Health, in its Final Report in 1961 (389), stated that:

> 'repeated exposure of the shameful, dehumanized condition of the mentally sick people who populate the back wards of State hospitals does not arouse the public to seek sweeping humanitarian reforms. . . . It has been the special view of the mental health professions that people should understand and accept the mentally ill and do something about their plight. The public has not been generally moved by this protest. People do feel sorry for the mentally ill, but in the balance, they do not feel as sorry as they do relieved to have out of the way persons whose behaviour disturbs and offends them. . . . The fact that society tends to reject the mentally ill is, of course, well known; little significance seems to have been attached to it, however.'

To take another example, it is interesting to note that, in Peru, where there is a relatively high prevalence of convulsive disorders, the general population show 'frank cultural rejection of epileptics' (63). But in England (where the prevalence of epilepsy is appreciably lower) it has been similarly recorded that:

> 'The public have long cherished the belief that epilepsy is synonymous with mental deficiency and uncontrollable criminal impulses . . ., and the epileptic is thus too often treated as a pariah. . . . Another unhappy outcome of the general ignorance and misrepresentation of epilepsy is the sense of guilt which it kindles in the parents, and which unless they are reassured may lead through mutual reproach to domestic strife, which reacts adversely on the child' (330).

Parallel with changes in popular attitudes to mental illness, there is a much more widespread realization, in many countries, of the comparatively high prevalence rates for mental illness that are found all over the world. Krapf and Moser (5) found that, of the countries which responded to their inquiry, in those where there were more developed hospital services the mentally ill occupied 40 to 50 per cent of all available beds, whereas in those where the turnover was slow they accounted for only about 2 to 3 per cent of all hospital admissions. These observers also remarked that where treatment methods were tending to increase the number of patients discharged as improved, there was a tendency for the hospitals to lose their stigma; thus patients would seek treatment voluntarily and at an earlier stage in the disorder, and had a greater chance of earlier return to the community. They suggested that it could be a healthy sign in a community when admission figures to mental hospitals tended to rise but hospital population figures tended to decline. Krapf and Moser also found that studies of the prevalence of mental illness have been extended beyond the hospitals. Some such studies (105) were carried out before 1948, but only in the last decade have attempts been made to estimate the numbers of mentally ill in large areas (109, 127).

Many observers have investigated the incidence of neuroses and the less serious forms of mental disorder, and have come to the general conclusion that the extent of these conditions is much greater than that of the psychoses. Various estimates have been made of the prevalence of these less serious conditions, ranging from 10 to 30 per cent of the population; but without standardized criteria and nomenclature it is hardly possible to make comparisons.

The view was expressed that, at least in the United States and probably in a number of other countries, there had, in the past twelve years, been a much greater acceptance by ordinary people of mental health services; that the prestige of mental health specialists, psychiatrists, and others had risen, and opportunities for careers in the general areas of mental health had multiplied. In those countries where funds are available for research, the amount of work undertaken in the field of mental health has increased. These trends suggest a much greater readiness to accept mental illness as an illness and not as something to be ashamed of. There are probably very striking differences in the strength of these trends, respectively, between individuals, between various groups in the community, and between social classes and ethnic groups.

The Study Group drew attention to important trends in many countries towards an increasing association between psychiatry, medicine, and surgery; towards the increased use of psychiatric concepts in other branches of medicine; and towards earlier referrals for psychiatric treatment.

A psychiatrist in the public health service cited, as an example of the greater involvement of citizens in some sort of service for people suffering from mental ill health, the state of Victoria, Australia, where, through various welfare organizations, an estimated half a million people out of a population of three million are personally concerned in some aspect of helping the mental health programme. In addition, there is a developing insight into mental health problems in everyday life, particularly among teachers, the clergy, public health nurses, child welfare authorities, and the staff of children's institutions. Youth leaders, and such organizations as the Young Women's Christian Association, Rotary, the Country Women's Associations, the Marriage Guidance Council, and so on, are tending more and more consciously to take part in mental health services in ways scarcely conceivable in the immediate postwar period.

The example of Victoria can be paralleled in a number of other countries, where, in addition, a new outlook on psychiatry is making an enormous difference to the work satisfactions of members of mental hospital staffs who were previously engaged only in custodial work.

Over the period since 1948 there has been a considerable increase in exchange of information and movement of mental health personnel across national and cultural frontiers. One of the most beneficial results has been a clearer appreciation that wide differences exist in attitudes towards mental illness and the mentally sick, among people of different cultures or social environments. There is now greater recognition of the fact that such diverse attitudes may, variously, help or hinder mental health work, and that their existence must be taken into account.

It is of the greatest importance that international bodies, and particularly the World Health Organization, should continue to promote and encourage these trends as they spread across national boundaries, not only by purely technical undertakings, but also in the field of communication and by developing techniques that foster good human relations between the many and various kinds of health worker.

CHANGING CONCEPTS OF MENTAL HEALTH

Up to now public concern for health, including mental health, has been mainly with disease, its treatment and prevention, and to a far less extent with the establishment of the best attainable state of health. Since World War II, though much still remains to be done in the way of helping the mentally sick and the handicapped, increasing understanding of the nature of tensions, anxiety, and social stresses that cause suffering, of inadequacy, and so on, has enabled workers for mental health to widen their horizons, to include these largely psychologically determined disturbances within their ambit and seek to prevent them. Great lacunae exist in our understanding of these matters but it is clear that success in tackling them requires the combined skills of many types of professional worker, with the backing of non-professional people and governmental action at times, nationally and internationally.

The modern concept of mental health which has been derived from the creative thinking of the last two generations pays attention to the quality of living, its creativity and productiveness, and to the individual's ability to withstand the stresses and strains inherent in living. In 1948, *Mental Health and World Citizenship* (12) included the remark (p. 25):

> 'The fact that men and women everywhere are looking for guidance in world affairs as well as in dealing with the problems in their own community, constitutes the greatest challenge ever presented to social scientists and psychiatrists.'

Before such a 'challenge' can be taken up, however, the role of the social sciences and psychiatry in world affairs needs more precise definition. It is now held by many that the tendency of these disciplines to enter the field of human welfare in a general capacity should not be encouraged.

A more fruitful approach, which has as yet been found in only very few places, would be for the social sciences and psychiatry to contribute specifically from their respective areas of competence to human welfare. In the words of an anthropologist in the Study Group:

> 'We could then take our knowledge of psychosis and neurosis, of character development, of the effect of drugs, of malnutrition, of disease, of institutional pressures on individuals, and of the way individuals distort institutions, and apply these aspects of professional competence, as appropriate, to a wide range of human problems.'

Let us take as an illustration the case of an individual child who has a very high degree of mathematical ability but who, in other respects, especially in the realm of human relations, is solitary and difficult to live with. He becomes isolated, rejected, and develops certain disagreeable reactive behaviour patterns. This not uncommon condition encountered in clinical practice might be regarded as a mental health problem in respect of which psychiatrists had a major degree of competence. But such a comparatively simple case presents related problems of consequence for society. For example, how to teach mathematics to this child so that society can enjoy the full value of his ability is a question for educationalists to consider; and the establishment of schools for the special education of children with unusual needs presents economic and social issues.

To take another illustration, this time from the wider sphere of world affairs: it would be reasonable in the interests of mental health for the social sciences and psychiatry to enter the discussion of problems of disarmament by contributing psychiatric and sociological knowledge of anxiety and the pathological aspects of fear. Thus, at the international political level, an attempt could be made to spread greater understanding of the nature of anxiety and fear between nations, of the effect of propaganda, and so on. In these kinds of way, the social sciences and psychiatry can offer their competence in dealing with individual and group, social and psychological difficulties towards the solution of the problems in human relations that are facing mankind.

THE CREATION OF A FAVOURABLE CLIMATE FOR GROWTH AND DEVELOPMENT

In the consideration of factors that influence growth and development, there has been a steady shift of emphasis away from the concept of the traumatic experience and its consequences, to a study of the opposite aspect – the effect on the child of a strengthening, facilitating type of experience. Unhappily for advances in knowledge, no generally accepted method has been devised of evaluating the effectiveness of those mental health measures that have been designed as strengthening and facilitating factors, although there are current developments in this respect.

Another new orientation, the importance of which cannot yet be fully appreciated, has taken place in the field of university education. The point was made in the Study Group that, traditionally, university education, especially in the field of the humanities, has been based on the triad of the teacher, the student, and the book. With the addition of the physical sciences to the university curriculum, the laboratory has tended to some extent to supplant the book. Medical education, which has developed largely outside strict university precincts, has for a long time included a fourth person in the teaching situation, namely, the patient, and this additional party is no less essential to psychiatric than to other aspects of medical education. A similar method of training has been spreading very widely among the other human sciences. The effect of the change of attitude involved can be seen in the kind of work that trained social scientists are now taking up; for example, it is estimated that in the USA 13 per cent of all the anthropologists in the field are working in mental hospital and psychiatric settings rather than in universities. Whereas in general medicine and psychiatry, and their related spheres, the fourth party in the training situation is the patient, in education the schoolchild is to an increasing degree being included with the student and the teacher as an active factor in the teaching process; and in the field of human relations in industry, the fourth party is the plant personnel. We might extend our example to the field of technical assistance to an underdeveloped country, and add that the governments and the technical assistance personnel can find the fourth party in the people of the country concerned.

The essence of this kind of training for students in the human sciences is that, instead of their learning opportunities being limited to books and lectures, they are now able to share in their teachers' knowledge of the relevant groups of human beings.

The comment was made that many people regard mental health as a new subject, as it were, which has somehow to be included, for example, in programmes of training of teachers. Our opinion is that mental health considerations are not in any way separable from those of education, which, being concerned with the conditions for optimum development, are impregnated in every aspect with mental health values. Just as the psychiatrist is concerned with facilitating the capacity of deprived or handicapped people to enjoy and participate in their humanity, so are members of other professions engaged in mental health work closely concerned with how the people with whom they are dealing are living their lives as human beings. From such a basis we may eventually be able to approach the larger questions that involve the state of the world.

Much more study is needed of the changing cultural conditions that can be found where one-time simple societies are exposed to modern technology. A social psychologist reminded the Study Group that social change, in Africa for example, as it occurs in indigenous populations, generally means a change in, a weakening or disappearance of, tribal institutions, economic structures, patterns of interpersonal relations, value systems, and cosmology. But the social change does not necessarily mean that tribal distinctions cease to be relevant for everyday life, for they may, in fact, promote solidarity in new social contexts, provide demarcation lines for political groupings, or form a basis for economic cooperation and rivalry.

However, it could not be disputed that the cultural concomitants of tribal life – the self-contained, equilibrated social systems – are often the first casualties of the changes that accompany the disturbance of a subsistence economy, of its village and community life, during the course of industrialization and urbanization. The changes that occur are sometimes regarded as acculturation, using this term in the sense of gradual assimilation to the culture of the so-called 'West'. It may not always be realized that the breakdown of traditional cultures may be followed by a period of cultural confusion and instability when little is institutionalized and when individual impulse tends to be dominant. When stability is re-established, the new cultures that emerge from such states of confusion may not be wholly along Western lines, and it is important to study the unique characteristics of such emerging cultures and their potential influence on the personality development of the individuals concerned.

In peasant cultures there have always been rigid limits to what people expect for themselves in the future; but at the Study Group an anthropologist remarked on the extent of the change in expectations that people are now entertaining for themselves, particularly in the less developed parts of the world. Perhaps not unconnected with these heightened expectations, technical assistance and other measures are now making very rapid change more possible in the newly developing countries. Hitherto, it has generally been considered that rapid change carries greater hazards for mental health than the slower processes of modification that extend over generations. However, during the period under discussion, there has been accumulated considerable understanding of change, introduced by many different agencies, and experienced on a massive national scale as in mainland China. Anthropologists have also carried out follow-up studies of communities known through previous work, and there has been intensive examination of nativistic cults and revitalization movements. Evidence is suggestive that processes of slow evolution are not necessarily the least stressful ways of change. There are a growing number of examples of successful passage, in the course of a single generation, from a peasant culture, in which personal expectations have been restricted to the traditional and only type of life the people know about, to a modern industrial type of community. The key to successful rapid change appears to lie in the altered expectations that people have for themselves and for the community as a whole.

CONCEPTS OF MENTAL HEALTH IN DIFFERENT CULTURES

In recent years it has become more widely recognized that the concept of mental health may have very different meanings for different people. The Federation has contributed to this realization through its international seminars and through its cross-cultural studies. The second study, *Mental Health and Value Systems: An inquiry into the compatibility of contemporary mental health concepts with various religions and ideologies* (41), was partly motivated by an awareness that, whereas the impetus towards spreading modern mental health concepts has come mainly from Western Europe and North America, many countries have been involved which, in history and tradition, are remote from the Judeo-Christian view of human nature and the good life.

In some parts of the world and particularly in Africa, instead of being dependent on the aid of scientific and experimental psychology, modern mental health activity has tended to be caught up in the traditional association of medicine and magic. In a society in which a man might run into the bush, believing that he was under the influence of witchcraft, and where his disturbed behaviour might be regarded by a modern psychiatrist as pathological, an immediate mental health function might be the promotion of 'white magic' or, in other words, the harnessing of superstitious belief in the supernatural for the welfare of the community. At the other extreme, the emphasis on a scientific approach to psychology that has marked much mental health work in Western European and North American countries has increased since 1948, even to the extent that doubt has been thrown upon the justification of any psychotherapeutic endeavour in the absence of statistical proof of efficacy.

Scientific interest in mental health has itself been moving in two separate directions: towards a better understanding of the physiology and biochemistry of the brain; and towards the study of behaviour, including animal behaviour, and psychodynamics. Possible ways of linking these two lines of development are now being opened up.

The Federation's study of mental health and value systems has reflected a resurgence of interest in values that is being expressed in many different forms, whether by increasing recognition of the connexion between religion and mental health, or by the appreciation of the paramount importance of his value system to the individual concerned. More than twenty years ago the late Susan Isaacs wrote of the role of the psychotherapist: 'We do not seek to mould the patient according to our views of what he should be like, but only for him to make his own changes in himself by understanding his own deeper wishes and counter wishes.' In our view, the mental health worker may be regarded as having a therapeutic role within the community, and, since the therapist is a ready recipient of negative and positive feelings and projections, his position must be made clear.

The moral role of the therapist, or the physician, or the mental health worker is inescapable, and, as a member of the Study Group remarked, 'It is sheer self-deception for him to suppose that he is not espoused to a particular moral system'. The notion that science does not involve values has been discredited for many years. Scientific values may not coincide with moral values, but science cannot be morally neutral; it depends for its existence on the appreciation of certain values, such as truth, for example. Furthermore, the mental health worker, therapist, or educator who is committed to an ethic in dealing with individuals does not leave this behind him when operating in the social and political sphere.

A strong body of opinion today holds that at the centre of mental health action should be the endeavour to diminish what Robert Burns described as 'man's inhumanity to man', and to increase the capacity of human beings to include all other human beings within their own genuinely accepted category of human. These appear to be basic values at a political level to which those concerned with mental health are committed.

We may attempt to sum up the change of climate of opinion with the remark that mental health is not so much concerned to show the way to a better world as to help people on the way, which latter task, in our view, might more acceptably be described as 'the greatest challenge ever presented' to human scientists concerned with this particular order of problems (cf. p. 63 above). The disturbance that mental illness must make in people's functioning, and, short of mental illness, some of the many psychodynamic mechanisms of a pathological order to be found in society, constitute a major part of this 'challenge'.

The difficulty of sharply defining the area of competence of the mental health worker may be illustrated by reference to bereavement. Whereas there are 'normal' and socially acceptable manifestations of grief, some aspects of mourning may resemble behaviour associated with pathological depression. In a thought-provoking paper, Engel (674) listed symptoms of grief for comparison with similar manifestations that are obviously within the realm of psychiatry, and therefore of medicine. Where the resemblance between grief and psychopathological behaviour is strong it would be logical to inquire whether mourning should not be regarded as pre-eminently a medical problem. This illustrative question is all the more pertinent because, as studies of grief and mourning in infancy by Bowlby (653–5) have demonstrated, grief in babies can have a very serious medical significance.

It is unreasonable to attempt to resolve in a brief discussion the question of what constitutes a medical or, more relevant in this context, a mental health problem. This is partly because these questions are extremely complicated, but more importantly because of a current lack of knowledge of how to differentiate sharply between the limited number of possible variations of human behaviour which, in different combinations, can have, respectively, some medico-pathological and some socio-normal significance.

6

Transnational Mental Health Problems

SOME RECENT DIFFICULTIES

The general tenor of information about mental health work in countries in which there has been any considerable degree of activity is that a fuller awareness of the implications of mental health action is spreading among ordinary citizens. However, along with growing awareness and improved understanding, there is also much misapprehension, to the extent that the difficulties of communication in this field in themselves constitute a formidable impediment to successful action.

It is very important that the growing body of knowledge of psychiatry and mental health action be more readily at the disposal of ordinary people, freed from its aura of mystery and from the anxiety-raising stigmata that have almost everywhere attached to the phenomena of mental illness. It may be useful to consider here some of the less rational reactions to mental health activities that are encountered, and more particularly their international or intercultural aspects.

First, there are some reactions, perhaps more or less universal, that are derived from the unique position of the physician in society. In the course of medical work there are circumstances, inevitably, in which the physician arouses both strong hopes and great anxieties in the people with whom he comes in contact. Throughout history the physician has been credited in popular imagination with both the power to cure and the power to kill. Modern advances in knowledge have resulted in the power to kill being largely separated from the power to cure, and these potentialities are no longer represented in the same person; but a fully parallel change has not necessarily taken place in the attitude of people towards the doctor.

The psychiatrist, as distinct from the physician or surgeon, is endowed by popular fantasy with those added qualities of mysteriousness that dealing with the mind appears to give, perhaps with powers that are more magical even than those of the miracle drug and the wonder operation; or more lethal than an error of prescription or a surgical operation that unexpectedly ends fatally. In addition, the psychiatrist must tolerate some of the consequences of being able to bring about change in his patients' behaviour. The patient who goes into treatment manifestly strange or even mad, and comes out sane, may appear to the ordinary onlooker to have been subjected to some mysterious but powerful influences, and the spectator may wonder whether such powers might conceivably be employed also to make sane people mad. The unscrupulous psychiatrist who uses his power of changing other people to gain his own selfish ends is a well-known character of sensational fiction. Religious and political history, and the history of witchcraft and sorcery in the community, show that those who are credited with powers of changing other people's attitudes are potentially in a very vulnerable position in society unless they are protected by the strong sanction of religious acceptance or political support.

Psychiatrists are accustomed on the most neutral social occasions to being met with remarks such as: 'I suppose you can read my mind.' Many cartoonists have drawn variations on the theme of two psychiatrists meeting, and one saying, 'Good morning. You're all right. How am I?' From such ascriptions of magical powers of mind-reading it is a logical step to ascribe powers of influence, also. A member of the Study Group recalled that when he was serving as a military psychiatrist a senior general used at one time to start official conversations with the remark: 'Don't you try to psycho-analyse me.' Although increasing confidence changed this conversational gambit into a ritual pleasantry, its origin undoubtedly had been defensive. A similar defensive mechanism can be seen in the origin of such playfully denigrating but affectively laden epithets as 'head shrinkers' and 'trick cyclists'.

It should not occasion surprise if the suspicion and fear which tend to become attached to the work of individual psychiatrists should also involve organizations in which psychiatrists have positions of influence. There may be some exacerbation of such attitudes in the not uncommon case of psychiatry and psychiatrists being not fully acceptable to the culture. Some indication of lack of acceptance may be seen in Great Britain, for example, in the use, until quite recently, of the term 'alienist' for a psychiatrist working in the field of mental illness – literally 'one who takes away from (society)'. In Great Britain, at least, and it may well be true of other English-speaking countries too, the psychiatric joke or cartoon is unfailingly popular, but it is a commonplace, if not a general rule, that the psychiatrist is presented as significantly deviating from the stereotype of the 'Anglo-Saxon', in appearance and language, and often remote, in a humourless way, from the foibles of the ordinary person. In some ways, the recent popularity of so-called 'sick' humour may represent a wider acceptance of psychiatric concepts. It would be interesting and informative to make some systematic studies of the place of psychiatry in humour, in a number of cultures.

Our concern here is with the likelihood that when psychiatrists are identified as foreign, to some extent, in the eyes of the ordinary citizen, mental health action will tend to have attached to it some of the attitudes – including the hostile aspects – that belong to foreign groups or concepts. This is a matter of considerable significance now that mental health action is so frequently crossing frontiers. It may get caught up in difficulties that are more strictly of a political nature. For example, in recent years there has been an additional source of embarrassment in that the role of the psychotherapist has, to some extent and in some places, tended to become confused in some people's minds with the attempt to change political attitudes by so-called 'brainwashing'.

It was remarked in *Mental Health and Value Systems* (41) that brainwashing is a term that has been coined in a pejorative sense, to describe a process of attitude change that is thought to be inimical to oneself or to one's own party or interests. Thus, the individual who changes from 'our side' to that of the enemy is a traitor, of whom the kindest thing that can be said is that he has been 'brainwashed' by the enemy; whereas he who changes from the enemy to our side may be thought to have been converted, or in some other way to have seen his former error.

These are some of the factors that need to be taken into consideration in any attempt to improve the mental health of people that involves a programme of advocating change, including change of attitude. It appeared to the Study Group that these complex questions of brainwashing, conversion, and change of attitude, with the attendant anxieties, fears, and hopes that may be aroused, can be of first importance to those who take on mental health work. It would be wise, if possible, to avoid adding the active opposition that may be engendered by displaced hostile attitudes to the personal and conceptual difficulties that will almost inevitably be encountered. An articulate minority in a community that regards a mental health organization as dangerous and threatening could stifle support and cripple fund-raising efforts, and there appears to be evidence of increasing articulate opposition in some countries. We should like to know of instances of a mental health organization successfully countering such opposition by the application of knowledge derived from the social and human sciences and from psychiatry to the problem of dealing with a hostile group. For example, to what extent has there been success in applying mental health principles to deal with groups of paranoid people in a community (who might be recognized under a term such as 'crackpots', and who might operate both in the open and also under the guise of organizations set up to preserve certain traditional positions from all innovation)?

Whereas in most places where opposition of this nature is encountered it is inspired by a local personality, or is more or less unorganized, there have been reports, particularly in the United States, of instances of local opposition from more highly organized groups of 'crackpots'. It appears that such opposition is likely to be chauvinistic or xenophobic, opposing mental health action on the grounds of conflict with values and attitudes that are traditionally dear to the society.

These are difficult issues and carry with them a considerable load of anxiety. The Study Group was itself conscious of a certain reluctance and some division of opinion among its members about the justification and wisdom of including an account of the discussion of these matters in this volume. However, after careful consideration of the various representations made by members, the editors have assumed responsibility for including what follows.

It appears that criticisms of and attacks on mental health activities tend to fall into one of three main divisions:

(i) accusations of brainwashing;
(ii) accusations of advocacy of change thought to be subversive (no single political ideology appears to have a monopoly of making this criticism);
(iii) the charge, implied contemptuously, of what has been termed, colloquially, 'do-gooding'.

The members of the Study Group were unanimous in their feeling that it is neither practicable nor justifiable merely to regard such attacks as deplorable and the people making them as stupid; nor to adopt an attitude of olympian certitude, which some people in the mental health field are alleged to do. It is perhaps even more unfortunate if an attempt is made by mental health workers, as sometimes happens, to interpret every criticism in terms of the critic's own motivations, without any consideration of the possible objectivity of the complaints that are made.

First, whether or not an accusation of brainwashing is made may, as remarked above, depend upon the critic's own identifications – whether he believes that a question of 'side' or party is involved. Second, the accusation that mental health workers engage in subversive activities may be hardly less subjective and is likely to follow from the former, or vice versa. There is a basic principle involved here – that mental health workers should aim to meet such challenges at their origin by applying their scientific knowledge to the situation. For example, the Study Group was informed of an instance of a nation-wide mental health organization with a federal structure that was threatened with the resignation of one of its member bodies on the grounds of the unacceptable political sympathies of some of its leading figures at the national level. The reaction of the organization was to examine the records of its employees ostensibly in order to verify whether the complaint was objectively based. Because they feared that there was a further intention of dismissing any employees who were found to be offenders, some people interested in the organization severely criticized this action at the time, on the grounds of moral cowardice. It appeared to the Study Group that yet another point of view might be argued: i.e. that the matter was no more than a technicality which had somehow been mistakenly elevated to the level of a moral issue; and that the best strategy for the national mental health organization in this instance would have been to apply technical skill to the problem at the level of its origin. In other words, it would have been better to seek to understand the motivation of the member body in bringing the objection, than to take action at the immediate manifest level of the problem.

Thirdly, the question of 'do-gooding' is a vexed one to which further reference will be made below. It can be argued that whether this question causes difficulty or not depends on whether mental health action is regarded as a 'movement'. There can be little doubt that an influential proportion of people interested in mental health work do, in fact, regard it in some such light, and it cannot be asserted that the field of action for mental health is free from proselytizing activity and claims. Undoubtedly some people in 'mental health' sometimes behave as if there is a resemblance between mental health and a religious system or a set of moral values. To them it is something in which they believe and which they wish their friends and neighbours to accept. Although such attitudes are not an essential part of mental health work and, indeed, are deplored by many, they cannot be entirely excluded. The history of endeavour for the betterment of mankind suggests that the motivation of those who take part cannot be sharply distinguished from that of the people who propagate religious causes.

When responsibly-minded people have confidence in a certain system it is understandable that they should seek to widen its application, and there are those who argue that mental health principles are useful not only in the prevention of mental ill health but also in the solution of social problems over a wide range, from the abolition of war to the increasing of the sum of human happiness. The application of a set of principles to the solution of problems of human society and human happiness is likely to lead people into self-determined activities which they may conceive to be in the interests of other people, and into making judgements on what they conceive to be the situation of other people. From this it is a short step to take action to alter that situation, with or without the consent and understanding of the people concerned.

It is desirable to maintain a proper perspective on mental health activity. It is hardly reasonable merely to dismiss it as unjustified interference, or social imperialism, or 'do-gooding', or whatever term of abuse is favoured. The motives and actions complained of in these strictures are perhaps the mainsprings of much work for human welfare, and to dismiss them with contempt is also to dismiss a major part of human altruism and unselfish action. However, it cannot be denied that these self-determined activities have the great disadvantage that they tend to attract hostility, even or especially from those people for whose good the activity is intended. Such well-meant but ill-judged activity may be a powerful trigger of the opposition to mental health work that is encountered, in that it arouses partly irrational defences against attempts at attitude change by outside influences.

It seems particularly important for mental health workers not to lay themselves open to criticism based on misunderstanding of this nature, and it is very pressing that the criticisms that have been made should be responded to by more concerted attempts to understand the psychological situation that has created them, to deal with misconceptions, and to allow for irrational patterns of critical reaction.

More is known about the individual than the group aspects of attitude change, and far more about small groups than about whole nations undergoing change. At the same time it appears likely that there is a quite considerable body of knowledge about the changing of attitudes of individuals and small groups which, with care, is capable of being extrapolated to some degree to a community level.

It is commonly accepted today in so-called mental health circles that, in addition to seeking to apply technical knowledge and skill to understanding the psychological roots of attitudes hostile to mental health work, it is extremely important to remain strictly within the sphere of recognized professional competence, but to take action as necessary in quite explicit terms, while dealing with any misunderstanding that becomes apparent.

The Study Group had much sympathy with the view that in the period from 1945 to 1961 an appreciable amount of mental health work had been vitiated by a failure to keep the boundaries of competence clearly in mind. This observation is particularly applicable to mental health action in the international sphere, where we have failed in many cases to make it clear to our critics that we seek only to apply mental health principles where they are valid, fully accepting that there are many areas in which we have no competence. For example, in the meetings involving diplomats that have taken place, it has been said that undue pressure has been exerted on the people concerned. Though it would be futile to deny that some change of attitude is being sought in most mental health activities, this is only one aspect and not the whole story, which is far more concerned with the spreading of understanding of the psychological principles underlying attitude change.

The moment that psychiatry steps over the narrow confines of concern with mental disorder, its cure and direct prevention, into any form of less direct preventive activity, it necessarily becomes involved in social attitudes. In so doing it runs the risk of provoking hostile reactions, to the extent that, in some communities, mental health work or human welfare work in this area has not been possible, owing to the intense opposition that the prospect of consequent change attracts. It is a first essential in any mental health activity that the community in which it is attempted should have a relatively liberal atmosphere. That is, it must be possible for an individual or group to advocate a wide range of change of attitude and change of social behaviour without inevitable conflict with the civil or political power, which must itself be prepared to countenance change.

Where the prevailing atmosphere of a social group compels the individual to conform to a pattern of thinking established by a dominant influence, it may be very difficult indeed to establish a programme of mental health activity. Acceptance of new ideas introduced as a result of mental health activities may throw the individual into conflict with authority and cause tension that endangers his mental health; furthermore, the members of a society may be prevented from attaining optimum mental health by the imposition of restrictive conditions, involving political or social coercion which denies the individual the expression of his own sentiments (see also Volume II).

Where conditions are restrictive, the advocacy of change that threatens to disturb existing social attitudes is almost bound to stir up hostility, which, ostensibly, may be mainly due to projection on the part of members of the community, but which may also be provoked by interfering and critical attitudes among the mental health workers themselves – attitudes that are no less hostile to the existing community atmosphere than are those of the community to the mental health workers. This situation contributes very much to the difficulties of mental health work and may well make action impossible in a given society.

It is more usual that the atmosphere in the community is neither particularly liberal nor strongly illiberal in the sense used above, but the existence of quite small illiberal elements can impede mental health work, when their hostility becomes attached to what mental health workers are trying to do. In such an event, criticisms tend to be directed against mental health in a non-specific way. It is the field – the whole notion – of activity that is objected to, whether by criticism, argument, or ridicule, and not so much the actual specific activities of mental health organizations. Thus, it is 'the kind of people' that get mixed up with mental health work who are subjected to comment, and there may be a tendency for hostile political feeling to develop.

THE LEGITIMATE ROLE OF MENTAL HEALTH WORKERS

The Study Group took the view that the complex problem of the legitimate role of the mental health worker had been distorted and obscured by arguments and discussions about professional competence, and by the observation of strict conventions about limited professional roles. Although it is recognized almost everywhere that mental health is a social, cultural, and psychological complex and not just a medical question, it remains true that many people think that medicine has a central place in mental health work, with the other professions somewhere on the periphery.

This view might be regarded as the outcome of a cautious, orthodox, professional medical attitude to an important new field of work; a recognition of an increasing challenge to medical thinking that has been made by the tension, anxiety, and social disturbances of current life, which may lead to suffering, inadequacy, and many psychosocial symptoms. There has been intense pressure on all professional people working in mental health to widen their horizons and to seek to break through the barriers of current ignorance in order to alleviate, and if possible prevent, these disturbances in so far as they may be regarded as largely psychologically determined.

The question of professional competence in this field has a paradoxical aspect, because while there are serious lacunae in understanding which only combined skills can hope to fill, there is also a considerable and growing body of knowledge about human relations which is not sufficiently being applied to problems in the mental health sphere. To remedy this situation will require a bold interprofessional approach.

It was remarked that among many divergent viewpoints affecting this issue, two appear to have been in particular opposition: respectively, that genuine advances in the mental health field can be made only by better understanding of the physiology and biochemistry of the brain; and that real progress can be made only by studying behaviour and psychodynamics. Conflicting though these views may be, the Study Group considered that there are a number of unifying threads to be found, but that more immediately practical questions for professional personnel to consider are: (i) what unites us all; and (ii) what distinguishes us from one another, in terms of our particular professions and skills.

It was suggested that one thread that unites us might be expressed in terms of a continuum of concern for human welfare, which extends from morbidity and crippling illness on the one hand, to the enabling of the individual to live an effective, creative, happy life on the other. What distinguishes one profession from another is the mode of entry into the matters of concern. For example, the educator is less concerned than the psychiatrist with crippling illness, and the psychiatrist is less concerned than the educator with the happiness and creative development of the great majority of children. Yet each profession may, from time to time, and in certain circumstances, be deeply concerned with those matters that are at the heart of the other profession's concern.

It appeared to the Study Group that the understanding of the role of mental health workers has been confused in some countries by a controversy that arose a decade or so ago between those who adopted a somewhat narrow attitude towards their professional role and those who felt a moral obligation to attempt to break through barriers of present ignorance in order to work towards the solution of problems of human wellbeing. In a presidential address entitled 'Psychiatry Ltd' to the Section of Psychiatry, Royal Society of Medicine, United Kingdom, in 1952 (670), Desmond Curran questioned the competence of psychiatrists to work in any area outside the narrow sphere of the treatment of mental illness. In contrast, many psychiatrists and members of other professions, including almost all those who support the work of WFMH and mental health organizations generally, hold the view that psychiatrists have a duty to apply their clinical experience to a wide range of social and psychological problems. But those who hold the latter opinion have not always recognized the obligation to enlarge their professional competence so as to enable them to operate efficiently with members of collaborating professional disciplines in preventive action in the social sphere. In other words, mental health must itself attend to the process of establishing its own professional discipline to which many existing professional disciplines can contribute.

The Study Group agreed that technical competence, though a fundamental requirement, is not the only criterion of professional excellence, and that acceptance of the moral commitment of the professional man to do what he can for human good may be equally, if not more, valuable. But it was also agreed that the professional man who accepts the moral duty to apply his skills for human welfare is under a moral compulsion to acquire competence sufficient to enable him to take on wider responsibilities. It appeared to the Study Group that the question of competence to do so is the central point of the controversy about whether the mental health worker should become involved in a programme of wide social action.

An educationalist member of the Study Group observed that some of the difficulties facing mental health workers arise from an uneasiness about accepting the fact of positive motivation for their work. He drew attention to the remarkable infrequency with which the word 'love' is used in connexion with mental health, and suggested that failure to admit the positive aspects of motivation may be a serious cause of uncertainty and vulnerability to criticisms.[1] We need also to consider the moral issues involved, for the concept of a science indifferent to values

[1] 'Love is Nature's second sun, bringing a spring of virtues where he shines.' George Chapman (1559–1634), *All Fools*, Act I, Scene I.

makes no sense in the sphere of human relations. Although it is one aspect of modern thought to make a distinction between ethics and politics, the values inherent in human relations make it imperative that the professional person operating in the political sphere be not divorced from his ethical position. The Study Group thought that in discussing two of the principal goals of mental health work – the diminution of man's inhumanity to man and the promotion of an increased capacity of human beings to include other human beings within the category of human – two of the basic values at a political level to which mental health workers are committed had been broached.

Quite apart from the moral issues involved, the Study Group considered that it is not justified automatically to assume that when psychiatrists concern themselves with human relations in connexion with mental health work, they must necessarily be outside the sphere of competence which they have a right to claim. Research into human relationships within small groups is now fairly well established, both in the context of industry and in that of the conference table. This research has been concerned with questions of leadership and the like, with the types of human relationship that obtain under conditions of stress, and with the effect that the composition of the group may itself have on the outcome of the group process.

It is reasonable to infer that mental health research knowledge about human relationships in small group discussions has an immediate relevance in the political sphere, for example, to meetings of leaders, at which decisions may be taken that could affect the destiny of nations. Another example in the political sphere of a legitimate interest of people concerned with mental health is the growing practice of interviewing politicians on television before an election. As a result, the politician may be tied down to follow a certain course of action if elected, because of a promise made in circumstances quite remote from the actual responsibilities he would then face. There is enough known about interview behaviour, for instance, to be of significant interest with regard to a political practice of this kind.

Study of the effects of cultural differences on the processes that go on in small groups has made a considerable contribution to knowledge of human relations, but the Study Group was at pains not to confuse the present state of knowledge with hopes and ambitions for the future. The Federation's activity must be based on current, not hoped-for future, mental health competence in the field of interpersonal relationships in small groups. Great care must be exercised in extrapolating this experience into the international field, recognizing the harm that might be done by ill-judged use of such material at the present time, in controversial international political issues.

A clear distinction must be made between carefulness to avoid involvement in political issues outside one's professional competence and the view of some people that it is not a proper aim of mental health work to bring about social change that is considered valuable. Any social change is likely to have repercussions in the sphere of political action, and it is impossible for people engaged in mental health action not to get involved to some extent even in highly controversial matters. For example, we have referred above to brainwashing, and have remarked that changes effected in human behaviour and attitudes may be regarded by some people as beneficial and by others as perverted or harmful. Which of these two attitudes is adopted towards social change taking place through mental health action may be determined by moral and ethical values as well as by political sympathy.

It cannot be other than disadvantageous for mental health action to be involved in political or social controversy, and it is vital that we should be more precise in public about our fields of competence. For example, it is generally agreed that we know more about small group functioning than about the functioning of vast societies; and that we are in a unique position to promote the transnational exchange of information concerning the mentally ill and methods of treatment, the social ill-effects of mental illness, the psychiatric aspects of technical change, and delinquency. Thus there is a great deal that we could say about these aspects of public welfare.

Those who are involved in mental health action not uncommonly get into difficulty through failure to realize that much of the criticism that they encounter is based on a false antithesis. For example, the proponents of 'psychiatry limited' seek to confine mental health action within the fields of proven scientific fact or generally accepted experience of psychiatry, and tend to imply that, if this is not done, the only possible alternative is 'mental health unlimited' – the application of mental health experience, without hesitation, in any situation, as a panacea. This is to equate 'mental health' with a movement of the order, say, of Moral Rearmament, which attempts to bring a single, universally applicable remedy to all situations. It is quite unreasonable to make a simple polar distinction between 'limited' and 'unlimited' as if there were no possibility of a middle way.

This is a key point that deserves further discussion, which will be introduced by an analogy drawn from an actual happening at the Study Group. At the beginning of one session the switchgear of the microphone failed, so that no tape record could be made. Neither a replacement of the faulty part nor the services of a skilled electrical engineer could be obtained within at least four hours, but it was considered highly desirable to record the discussion, to which the participants had travelled many thousands of miles. One member of the Study Group, equipped with a school knowledge of electricity and a training in medical examination and diagnosis, set out to detect and, if possible, remedy the fault, which he did successfully in half an hour.

No member of the Group, including the individual himself, had any confidence in the volunteer's competence to solve the problem; some thought that more harm than good would result from an unqualified person's interference with expensive equipment. The determining circumstance was that, by waiting for technical competence to be mobilized, the record of the discussion would have been lost beyond recapture. The volunteer took the view that the circumstances imposed an obligation to apply the best available skill with the greatest possible care, because the situation could not be remedied in any other way. It does not affect the principle that the volunteer succeeded, or that he was not quite clear at the end how he had done so. The essential points are that he could estimate the maximum extent of the damage that it was possible to inflict and that he took care in utilizing his knowledge of the principles of electricity to minimize the risk of doing harm; also, what was more important, he could apply his trained powers of observation and reasoning to the problem, and could be guided by his realization of his technical limitations.

It may be argued that the field of mental health often produces analogous situations. A difficult or dangerous situation may arise – individual or group – in which it is clear that, unless something is done, serious loss or disaster will follow. There may be no possibility of finding anyone with a proper level of technical competence in time to influence the course of events; but people may be available who have sufficient grasp of the principles necessary to deal with this or an analogous problem, and who realize their own technical limitations clearly enough to enable them to operate with safety, although their scientific knowledge may be very incomplete.

In recent years, Bowlby, Spitz, and others have produced evidence about the possible morbid effects of lasting separation of infants from their mothers (407–15, 653–55, 675). The validity of the evidence has been, and is still being, challenged on many grounds – both philosophical and scientific. On strictly scientific, and even on moral and ethical, grounds it may be agreed that much of the evidence is not entirely convincing, but there is a widespread impression that it is the best that is available. There are few people in Western Europe and North America, once they have become thoroughly familiar with the data, who are prepared to ignore them when faced with the problem of a young infant away from its mother. Little public criticism attaches to mental health workers who take action based on the hypothesis that has been put forward; on the contrary, there may be an outcry if this new knowledge is not applied, however scientifically uncertain it may be. Where the emotional cathexis is high, there is little opposition to measures that are taken in good faith by people who attempt to apply the best knowledge that they possess with due awareness of their own limitations. The strict canons of scientific research method are not the most powerful factors operating in this area.

We have discussed above some of the criticisms and difficulties that may face mental health workers as a result of the confused application of a supposed moral principle of strict scientific validity. The controversy about what some people have termed 'Bowlbyism' is a good example. However, the real point at issue in this instance is not the purity and validity of scientifically collected evidence. The moral principle involved here is the duty to take whatever steps are possible in an endeavour to prevent harm occurring to very young children, when there are reasonable grounds for the fear that harm might follow if such action were neglected.

Another example can be seen in the confusion of moral argument that is often heard on occasions when action is taken to coerce a non-volitional patient into psychiatric treatment. Few people, and psychiatrists less than most, would question the fundamental principle of safeguarding the rights of the individual. But, in practice, the decision whether or not to apply compulsion is based not so much on balancing an assessment of the patient's needs against human rights as upon the practicability of compelling treatment; that is, whether treatment facilities are available, and the means of getting the patient into treatment; and, above all, whether there is a medical conviction that treatment is the course of action most likely to benefit the sufferer.

The Study Group came to the conclusion that the question of whether or not to take some particular action in the interests of mental health can rarely, if ever, be decided on the principle of whether there is enough proven scientific knowledge to justify the action. Some of its members doubted whether there is any valid moral basis for such attitudes as that of 'psychiatry limited'. They took the view that to approach a situation in the light of a preconceived judgement as to a moral issue involved is probably to ignore the most significant relevant factors. Perhaps the critical question to ask repeatedly is whether enough is known to justify a certain course of action when it is evident that no other course holds any promise of a more hopeful outcome.

This admittedly pragmatic principle, of the best possible available action, is extremely relevant for application to the contemporary international scene in the mental health field. No community provides adequately even for the most serious mental illness among its members, let alone for the many other social, psychological, and educational problems that may arise. Mental health organizations, which exist in less than half the countries of the world, are everywhere confronted with an urgent situation. They are subjected to pressures to take action on inadequate technical information and often with primitive resources. In most countries, whether there is an organized mental health group or not, people are making some progress in the field, and this is a cause for some satisfaction, but nowhere is even an approximately adequate job being done.

7
Mental Health Action

APPRAISAL OF EFFORTS

Though the attempt must be made, it is extremely difficult to assess the effect of action in the field of mental health. For example, it is virtually impossible to answer even the simple question: What things have happened through the World Federation for Mental Health? No one organization or particular group of people can take all the credit for favourable happenings in this sphere, although it can be claimed with confidence that the Federation has played an active role in the development of a climate favourable for mental health progress. There is evidence in the Federation's records of new initiatives being undertaken in many parts of the world following upon conferences, meetings, and other activities: for example, the establishment in a country of an industrial mental hygiene service; or modernization of mental hospital outpatients' activities; interdisciplinary conferences for social welfare; the introduction of mental health principles to other social welfare organizations; and the appointment of mental health advisers to governmental and intergovernmental agencies. These and other similar activities can fairly be ascribed at various times and places to the efforts of the Federation and others concerned with mental health action. Though useful and satisfactory, such examples do not themselves provide conclusive evidence of worth-whileness of action, nor do they silence the criticisms of those many people who are dissatisfied with the present state of factual knowledge as a basis for mental health work.

One of the major difficulties in interpreting the aims of mental health work to the educated but non-professional public appears to have been a general failure to make an appropriate distinction between what has been established scientifically and what remains a matter of conjecture and opinion. Many people feel that mental health action has too much of the spirit of a 'movement' in the sense of a crusade, and that there is more readiness to preach out of emotional conviction than to undertake patient study for the elucidation of fact.

Mental health work is hampered both by the unscientific enthusiasm of its protagonists and by the equally uncontrolled prejudices of its opponents. Innumerable examples might be given of reasonable propositions for mental health action based on established knowledge that have been emotionally rejected by political or professional authority. Some of the most emotionally conditioned opposition to mental health action has come from the medical profession, but this experience is not unique to mental health: public health in its day has also had to contend with much irrational opposition from the medical profession as well as from the public.

RESEARCH AND COLLECTION OF INFORMATION

That there has been a great increase in scientific work at a high technical level is shown by the stream of publications and reports that is now forthcoming. In respect of the aetiology, treatment, and prevention of mental disorders, the application of epidemiological methods developed in the field of public health and communicable disease is proving remarkably fruitful. Appreciation of the necessity for multidisciplinary cooperation in scientific research is resulting in improved methods of publishing findings, and of indexing and sorting information; in the organization of seminars and conferences for the exchange of recent findings; and in national and international travel for the comparison of results.

The Study Group was impressed by the need for the development of new conceptual tools, but many research workers pay no more than lip service to this idea and succumb all too easily to the temptation to continue working with old ideas and procedures. One striking example of this is the tremendous weight still placed upon the method of controlled experiment and statistical evaluation of results. This conceptual export from the physical sciences is widely recognized to make only a limited contribution in the biological sphere and even less in the psychological. We can find no record of scientifically controlled experiment being successfully carried out in the field of mental health; and it may be suggested that no such experiment will be practically possible except on those rare and unwanted occasions when natural disasters, war, and other cataclysms may arbitrarily provide the experimenter, if he happens to be in a position to take action, with two sets of conditions which approximate to a controlled situation. The use of a control and the reduction of variables have proved more than elusive concepts in mental health studies. It seems probable that much promising research initiative is being frustrated and efforts stultified by inability to look beyond methods developed in the natural sciences to more appropriate *ad hoc* techniques.

These new ideas and methods that are necessary may be at various levels of technical complexity. For example, at the most complex level, the concept of mental health which was widely agreed in 1948, though now being extensively modified, still gives a conceptual basis to much activity in the mental health field, and in this way constitutes a 'tool' for use in research. Other more practical procedures are no less important; for example, the more clinical techniques of analysing patterns of functional failure, or of collecting data over a wide area and looking for patterns of interrelationship. An illustration of the latter is the study, by an industrial medical officer concerned with the mental health of workers on a production line, of the relationship between the symptomatology or other behavioural phenomena of the workers and the various stages of the working timetable. This simple method could be applied, under direction, by a factory foreman. Though crude, this device embodies an important new conceptual tool – to use the actual process that is being studied in the evaluation of its phenomena.

We would draw particular attention to three aspects of mental health research that, in our opinion, need more attention: first, the detection and analysis of errors committed by the research team, whether in appreciation of the situation or in practical action; second, the weakness in conceptualization of mental health itself (the 1948 concept is now thought to be out of date in many ways); and, third, the time that is required for the evaluation of processes, in regard both to the objects and to the processes of study.

Another aspect of fact-finding which is not adequately handled at present is making known to the educated public the information that is available. The Study Group considered that it is the duty of the scientist to take the initiative in presenting information to the public, provided that the possible implications of scientific progress are also brought to the people's attention. For example, in the case of nuclear energy, it is the duty of the scientist not only to inform members of the public about the social uses of nuclear power so that 'atoms' are no longer mystery and magic but an understood concept, but also to warn them of probable alterations of social conditions from an unlimited supply of cheap energy – the effect on the working patterns and economic life of the community, and so on. (The failure of scientists to inform the public of the damaging aspects of nuclear energy, and to make clear the scientists' own share in making possible the harnessing of nuclear energy to processes of destruction, is another vital social question, but not one that can be taken up for discussion here (532).)

Those concerned with mental health work have not only the scientific competence but also the moral imperative themselves to inform the public, rather than wait to be asked. We have remarked (p. 72 above) on the position of the physician, traditionally endowed in popular fantasy with the power both to cure and to kill, and have suggested that psychiatry, which is at the centre of mental health action, is to an even greater extent than medicine generally the source of both hope and anxiety to the people who come in contact with it. There are many worries and fears (we used the example of brainwashing) that tend to be caught up in the public image of psychiatry, and therefore of mental health. These complications do not absolve mental health workers from the responsibility of unceasingly attempting to present their information to the public – indeed, they increase the moral imperative to be active in this way.

In recent years a new factor has arisen in the processes of information-giving, because of the application to propaganda of methods derived from psychology. For example, so-called psychological warfare, deliberately developed during World War II, has come to occupy an important place in the anxieties and fantasies of the public in the field of politics, and influences hopes of peace and fears of war. It is a problem of current mental health work that the public image of the psychiatrist has to some extent become involved in such harmful and socially destructive popular notions.

Mental health work often meets with a difficulty in connexion with the traditional conceptual tool of 'truth', thought of as 'ultimate' or 'absolute', the search for which has been characteristic of philosophical religious systems throughout the ages. Many religious, ideological, and political groups have laid claim to possessing absolute truth and, explicitly or implicitly, have held all who do not agree to be in error.

It is increasingly realized that the concept of 'truth', or more precisely, of a single, ultimate, or absolute truth, is proving as elusive in the scientific world as it has proved during centuries of discussion of philosophy and religion. It may be argued that the proven empirical data of science can represent 'ultimate truth' only to the degree that they are related to all the factors and influences operating in the situation. As methods of investigation improve and instruments become more refined, what was previously taken as truth gives place to some more comprehensive assessment of phenomena.

The notion of ultimate truth has proved to be one of the great difficulties in dissemination of mental health information, especially in attempts to convey to a public educated in styles of thought traditional to the humanities and literature, and brought up in the principles of a revealed religion, the relative nature of mental health research data. Such difficulties may be expected to decrease with the spread of scientific education but, as many communities have already experienced, the spread of scientific sophistication is apt to disturb previously accepted religious and moral conventions and to cause disorientation which may bring other mental health problems in its train.

One of the most important new conceptual methods, as we have remarked, is that of interdisciplinary cooperation on a basis of equal opportunities to contribute. This involves a departure from traditional attitudes towards professional competence, and is the antithesis of the restrictive outlook of 'psychiatry limited'. When two people of different disciplines set out to communicate across the boundaries which separate them professionally, each must be prepared to operate across the frontier which, if it is not to join them together, must inevitably separate them. Without a degree of preparedness not only to use the frontier as a bridge but also to allow the other party to use it, no interdisciplinary cooperation is possible.

THE GOALS OF MENTAL HEALTH ACTION

During the period under review the visible goals of mental health action have been many and varied, and very few workers have shown the single-mindedness of the 1948 report: 'This, then, as we see it, is the ultimate goal of mental health, to help men to live with their fellows in one world.' Much mental health activity today could be epitomized by the statement that the ultimate goal of mental health action is to help men to live with their anxieties in a changing world. This is an urgent matter in a world in which the paramount need of mankind is to find a way of life that will not lead to mutual and universal extermination. The capacity of human beings to live with their own anxiety now has a vital significance not known in any previous generation.

Many people regard the single-minded aims of 1948 as unduly promoting uniformity, and they react adversely by criticizing what they regard as the excessive conformism of some mental health attitudes. In the words of a member of the Group, it is not a mental health objective that the poet, the protester, and the creative artist should disappear. Moreover, in social action across cultural boundaries, values from the culture of the worker may not be automatically applied to the field of work. The mental health worker abroad must not grind, and must avoid the appearance of grinding, his own ideological axe.

With increasing professionalization, mental health work is playing a big part in social programme-making, especially in the field of child welfare, and must therefore strictly avoid attachment to any particular ideology or political system. Where concerted social action is involved, there is a possibility that mental health may become, or at least be regarded as, something of a cult, in a pejorative sense of the word. It may well happen that certain values that have become inherent in mental health work in some part of the world may not be held in high regard in other places to which mental health work is spreading, with the result that there may be a tendency for mental health to be looked upon in the latter places as something of an esoteric cult. Such attitudes are unlikely to arise when mental health action is taken in the more desperate social situations, such as mass displacement of population, and the like. In these cases, and indeed whenever action is taken on a wide scale, it is generally advantageous for mental health measures to be introduced to people as part of, or an extension of, activities designed to promote general public health.

Among people concerned with mental health action there is a growing climate of opinion that their ambit should extend beyond these urgent though limited social problems, and include the vital problems of survival that are facing the world, especially the endeavour to transform into a reality the possibility of a world without war.

The emerging phenomena of psychological independence, both of individuals and of communities, are issues on which the disciplines that have to do with mental health can have much to say. Not only are great changes taking place in the life of all newly emerging and hitherto underdeveloped countries that have gained political independence since World War II, but also all over the world the radical alteration of old-established ways of life calls for qualities of individual self-reliance which have not been required among the majority of people in most parts of the world in earlier times.

This increasing concern with broader social issues has naturally led to a feeling on the part of some people that mental health is neglecting the true centre of its interests, conceived of as the care of the mentally ill and the mentally handicapped. In some places the most rapid developments in the field of action for mental health have taken place more or less out of touch with the institutional treatment of mental disorder or deficiency, and in these places a high value is set on the goal of taking therapeutic and preventive action into community and family life. Many people hold that the primary aim of mental health action in this connexion is, by the excellence of mental hospital work, to improve the interpretation of the concept of mental illness to non-professional people in order to secure increasing public support of institutional mental health care. Others hold that it is not the primary concern in mental health to improve mental hospital services, but rather to improve community attitudes by more direct educational methods so that the hospitals can have the moral and financial support necessary to set their own house in order. However, the quality of much mental health activity depends upon the effectiveness of research into the aetiology and pathology of mental disorders, so that there may well be a growing but paradoxical tendency for mental health action to become relatively less involved with the community and relatively more, once again, with the problems of mental illness.

Notwithstanding modern research trends, it is being increasingly realized that the problems of the mentally ill and the mentally handicapped overlap all along the line with other living problems of individuals: their adjustment to work, family life, involution, and, especially, old age.

The psychiatric problems of old age have become an important mental health concern, as illustrated, among many other studies, in a report from Newcastle, England, where, although the proportion of over-65s in institutions was found to be not higher than 5 per cent, some 40 per cent of a random sample of over-65s had significant psychiatric disorders, mainly reactive depression or anxiety (651).

This discussion topic would be incomplete without reference to the view held by many that there is no need for a precise definition of the goals of mental health action, that precision may be dangerous when, as sometimes happens, mental health principles that have been embraced with enthusiasm in some part of the world are applied uncritically elsewhere. According to this view, the most important function of the World Federation for Mental Health at the international level is to strengthen national mental health organizations and to promote new ones; and that of national mental health organizations is to stimulate activity at the local level.

RELIGION AND MENTAL HEALTH

Since 1948 considerable change has been seen with regard to the place that religion is occupying in mental health work, a change that in many countries is part of a wide movement bringing religion into close touch with social concern and health activities. It was remarked with some mild cynicism that apparently the shortest route to becoming a psychiatrist in some countries was first to become a clergyman or a social worker.

In the 1948 statement, specific encouragement was given to clergy and religious groups to be more active in the mental health field as an integral part of their work. It appears that the concept that body and mind constitute a continuum in relation to health and disease has spread to include the spirit. In the words of a member of the Group, the nature of a man's religion is related to his emotional and psychological health, and an individual may use his religion according to his psychological needs. One practical aspect has been the mutual recognition by clergy and mental health workers that the former have a valid professional role in relation to the latter.

In theological schools in the United States there has been an increase in active training in psychological principles, and in the provision of training and clinical experience in problems of emotional illness. Many theological students are now given an opportunity to work under supervision in mental hospitals. Numbers of churches in the United States have their own counselling services or centres. Some have clinics staffed by psychiatrists and psychologists, and many others arrange for the part-time services of a psychiatrist. It is estimated that some clergymen may spend as much as half of their time in counselling, a responsibility that may prove dangerous if the individual's training is inadequate.

Similar developments, though not to the same extent, are reported in the United Kingdom, where in more than half of the English dioceses the clergy now have an opportunity to join in groups studying clinical problems of mental illness. In theological colleges there is a movement gaining ground to give students experience in mental hospital work and in the study of personality. In many other parts of the world, the role of the clergy in mental hospitals and in the handling of serious problems of mental illness and disorder is being increasingly recognized.

SOCIAL ASPECTS OF MENTAL HEALTH ACTION

One of the most important of the modern shifts of emphasis in the relationships between psychology, sociology, and medicine has resulted from the application of principles developed in individual dynamic psychological studies to small group functioning. That this interaction of psychology, sociology, and anthropology is capable of illuminating psychiatry has been demonstrated by studies of the social organization of the mental hospital, and by the definition of the 'sick role' in different societies.

There has been a parallel trend towards incorporating more of the biological sciences in the studies of abnormal behaviour, e.g. biochemical genetics, psycho-pharmacology, physiology, etc. The application of social disciplines, including cybernetics, as well as psychiatry to the understanding of community psychiatric problems has added to the individual approach of the psycho-analyst some newly developing sociotherapeutic skills geared to larger numbers of people in need of help. The change that is taking place can be illustrated by reference to *Mental Health and World Citizenship* (12):

> 'It is clear that no world-wide standards of mental health services can be set up since countries differ so much in economic resources and cultural setting. No general standards, universally applicable, can therefore be devised for providing a given number of psychiatric hospitals, clinics, etc., per unit of population. This question is simply part of the whole problem of correctly allocating the effort and often limited resources of a community for the common good.
>
> 'A society undergoing rapid change may readily accept principles of mental health in the construction of a new educational system or a public health plan, while societies which are already highly developed in these respects may actually be found more resistant. Illiteracy, simple levels of social organization and wide dispersion of population are not necessarily obstacles to the promotion of mental health principles. By the timely use of appropriate methods, it may be possible to avoid many of the evils which are found in the more industrialized societies' (p. 13).

These paragraphs continue to be largely relevant today, but in many respects we know more about the applicability to other countries of ideas or practices developed elsewhere. For example, in those countries that have long-established and highly developed mental health services, psychiatric hospitals, clinics, etc., there may be many practices that have become thoroughly institutionalized, which originated at an early stage in the country's development and have since been recognized as undesirable. The very large mental hospital dispensing prolonged custodial care is now seen to aggravate rather than diminish the patient's illness.

Single methods of therapy that make no allowances for individual variations may do more harm than good. Time-honoured practices in certain non-psychiatric fields, e.g. the handling of mothers in obstetric hospitals, or visiting rules in some children's hospitals, may be seen to have harmful mental health implications. Thus, as the quoted passage states, one effect of set institutional practice that has been developed at an earlier stage may be that the society in question is more resistant to innovation.

Though disadvantageous in the countries in which they occur, these set situations can be used to advantage as examples to prevent the same patterns being repeated in new developments in other countries, e.g. the tendency to disrupt the family in hospital childbirth; separation of mother and child; or long periods of impersonal institutional care for young children. The ex-Director-General of WHO, Dr Brock Chisholm, recounted how, some years ago, the doctor in charge of a new children's hospital ward in a West African country apologized for the fact that every inch of floor-space was taken up by members of the children's families camped out around the cots. He explained that no amount of persuasion could keep the families away. Dr Chisholm begged him not to try, and remarked on the enormous efforts now being made in Western Europe and North America to get the families back into the children's hospitals after their banishment three generations ago in the drive against sepsis and cross-infection. Why should this West African hospital go through a cycle of events bearing no relation to local conditions?

In planning new services at a modern residential nursery in Athens, it was possible to make full use of the contributions concerning infant care that have been made by René Spitz, John Bowlby, Jenny Aubry, and others, because key personnel of the project had attended the International Seminar on Mental Health and Infant Development organized by WFMH, in collaboration with WHO, UNESCO, and the Grant Foundation, at Chichester, England, in 1952 (510).

A member of the Study Group remarked that though it is essential to bring about a truly symbiotic development of ancient, familiar, and traditional institutions and modern scientific knowledge, there are certain dangers to be guarded against. Sometimes recent findings about the separation of infants from their mothers have been interpreted too literally or too rigidly. For example, there are cultures in which grandparents or fathers have more time available than the mother to be with the children, but a rigid interpretation of modern separation data may cause these potentially adequate mother-substitutes to be rejected. Elsewhere, emphasis may be laid not so much on continuity of adult-child relationship as on biological motherhood; or the mother may be required to leave her other small children at home in order to spend time at the hospital with the baby, although it may be that the father or a grandparent could on occasion provide relatively more adequately for the needs of the baby in hospital than for the remainder of the children at home.

Emphasis on the value of breast-feeding, which in many countries has arisen partly to counteract the overwhelming predominance of artificial feeding, has often been applied with more enthusiasm than discretion to feeding problems occurring during the period of transition from primitive or rural economies to urban life. Where breast-feeding is universally practised, the infant mortality rate is frequently high, and it is acknowledged that supplementary feeding should always be available, otherwise the mortality rate will remain high. In other countries, too, failure to recognize the biological origins of the anxiety that is commonly felt by the mother whose infant does not thrive on her breast has caused many mental health problems among the more educated and responsibly-minded mothers. It is now widely realized that even the most obvious principles need to be applied with caution and with due regard to local conditions.

In many countries, changes are taking place in public attitudes towards what is considered to be a 'social problem', or 'deviant behaviour', or 'mental disorder' in the particular culture. For instance, in England there have been several recent attempts, with varying degrees of success, to amend earlier legislation, and to introduce new and more enlightened laws, on such matters as prostitution and homosexuality (579), suicide and attempted suicide, therapeutic abortion, artificial insemination (550), and the treatment of offenders (478).

Public reactions to health programmes and their concomitant problems in various cultural and social environments are well illustrated by the case studies collected by Paul (645). For example, the very pressing question of fertility control remains unanswered, so far as the modification of particular cultural attitudes (546) is concerned, and in spite of the most promising developments of medical science in the production of steroid oral contraceptives (547). The problem is becoming of the utmost urgency to the populations of certain areas, e.g. Mauritius (508, 548, 549).

Mental health aspects of ageing have been discussed in many recent publications (306–7, 311–13). The social problems of the reciprocal attitudes of youth and old age, in connexion with juvenile delinquency and adolescent behaviour patterns, have been well summarized by Gibbens (318).

Some other aspects of contemporary society of particular concern for mental health have been increasingly studied in recent years: for example, the mental health, social, and cultural aspects of technical change (504, 520, 536); human problems presented by progress in industry and automation (471, 516–18, 522–25, 528–30); the mental health and social implications of industrialization and urbanization (520–21, 526–27, 531); and the mental health aspects of the peaceful uses of atomic energy (532).

Comparison of current attitudes in relation to industrialization with those of 1948 can be made by reference to the report of the Third International Congress on Mental Health (467). Attitude changes have been slight and progress no more than patchy. Jean Stoetzel used a particularly forward-looking phrase in the 1948 report: 'Social psychology as applied to industry will be unable to avoid the necessity of raising the question of values.' But although in 1961 some mental health workers might have a more serious attitude towards values, the meaning and moral significance of work remain obscure to the majority of workers, as they do to most scientific and technical writers.

A very considerable change has occurred in the direction of increased realization that, in this as in other fields of mental health effort, no single professional technique is sufficient by itself: that individual psychology alone is not sufficient for the understanding of group psychology; that social psychology is not sufficient in order to understand sociology; and that economic, political, and technological sociology lead sooner or later to questions of philosophy. Conversely, it is no less untenable that either a philosophical conception or a sociological theory can by itself explain individual or collective psychological phenomena.

ATTITUDES TOWARDS REALITY

Many writers have remarked upon the prevalence of apathetic attitudes towards dangers and difficulties facing society, and have regarded such group attitudes as analogous to psychotic withdrawal from reality and refusal to face problems. The Study Group thought that 'mental health' ought to have something to say about such reactions and their significance.

In the development of her more positive concept of mental health, Marie Jahoda (31) has included the notion that, in order to be mentally healthy, a person must have an adequately objective perception of reality. This proposition may be applicable to a wide range of current problems and concerns; one of the most urgent on the international plane, for example, is the whole question of attitudes towards other people of different racial or ethnic background. Any prejudice or stereotype about other people distorts the individual's perception of reality, since objectivity depends on adequate perception both of other people and of oneself. The individual who may perceive himself as superior to another individual because of the relatively light, or dark, colour of his skin has – if objectivity is taken into account – a distorted vision of himself, with consequences to himself potentially as severe as those from the distortion of his perception of the other person.

To the extent that the individual is bound by his own ethnocentric perception and nationalistic bias, he is prevented from seeing and understanding adequately and objectively the motives and attitudes of others in international relationships. This key concept can be illustrated negatively by consideration of the perception of the world and of himself by the mentally ill person, especially by one who suffers from a paranoid condition. The paranoiac views himself as the focal point of the chain of events that involve him; and his perception of all other people's actions is only in terms of relationship to himself, a situation that resembles the viewpoint of the ethnocentric individual.

It is a primary modern mental health concept that these aspects of interpersonal relations, whether on an individual, collective, or international level, must be examined in respect of prejudices and stereotypes, ethnic and national hostility, and racial discrimination; and in respect of the way in which these factors interfere with the individual's or group's capacity to reach an adequate level of objectivity of attitude and thus an optimal state of mental health.

A valuable experience of mental health action in the United States was reported to the Study Group, in which attention was drawn to a number of factors affecting the question of racial integration in schools in the Southern States. The report of the Group for the Advancement of Psychiatry (GAP) on *Psychological Aspects of School Desegregation* (572) helped to clarify the underlying issues in a number of communities confronted with this problem, but also aroused some hostility, perhaps because it revealed some unpalatable truths.

The concept of an adequate perception of reality that we have in mind is complex. More is involved than the attempt to achieve, or to substantiate a claim to, an undistorted perception. Perhaps the primary consideration is how far the individual can be aware, at least to a certain extent, and in some cases even to a large extent, of the distortions influencing his perception.

In evaluating the adequacy of an individual's perception of reality and insight into his own distortions of perception, the possibility of the presence of powerful psychological defences that may directly affect reality perception must be borne in mind. For example, at the end of 1945 it appeared to some observers in Berlin that some of the people who seemed the most mentally healthy showed the greatest indifference to the difficulties and dangers that surrounded them. These people were apparently getting on with their own work with a minimum of interference from anxieties and irrelevant pressures, were sleeping better, and were more buoyant in mood. They could have been regarded as living in a fool's paradise or, in other words, as showing a hysterical dis-association; or, at another level of personality integration, as showing apathy combined with a quality of resignation.

However, a third view could be taken – which may have more significance in terms of mental health – that these apparently mentally healthy people in Berlin had clearly perceived not only the full extent of the dangers and difficulties surrounding them but also the limitations of their own capacity to take effective action. It could be argued that, having assessed the situation as being outside their field of competence, they then controlled their anxiety, so that it should not interfere with their daily living. It is a tenable view that, in certain circumstances, the repression of anxiety arising out of a reality situation is no less healthy and no less necessary than the repression of anxiety arising out of the modification and control of instinctual drives which is demanded of individuals in order to live normally in society.

In other words, adequate perception of reality includes the realization that in certain circumstances nothing can be done about a situation. Since, to be mentally healthy, the individual requires the capacity to act in accordance with his perception of reality, he must be able to control his anxiety, however reasonable, so that it does not interfere unduly with his conscious activities.

It is essential for a community that both anxiety engendered among individuals by adequate perception of reality and anxiety raised by the modification and sublimation of instinctual drives should be effectively controlled. An illustration can be taken from current difficulties in inter-race relations in the Republic of South Africa. If a more adequate perception of the facts should result in all South African citizens becoming convinced that there was no essential significant difference between white and black citizens in respect of intellectual and other capacities, it would be logical to infer that this fresh perception would only increase the anxieties of the white citizens, who could then not escape the conclusion that it would be impossible to maintain their privileged position. It may be noted that the same conviction would be held from their standpoint by the black citizens. Similarly, if all the citizens came to recognize the fact that there is no logical or inherent connexion between a man's culture and his race, the white citizens would not rationally be able to maintain the notion that it is necessary for the mental health of all citizens that each should continue to pursue his own current cultural ways. Acknowledgement of these facts by all parties would bring the idea of an integrated society into the foreground, would challenge the government position in these matters, and, no doubt, greatly increase anxiety.

The traditional course of action in a conflict situation is to attempt to safeguard one's own security by adding to one's opponent's insecurity. There are innumerable instances of this pattern in the animal kingdom, and in terms of human behaviour examples are no less widespread. At the international level, recurrent armaments races illustrate the attempt of one side to make itself more secure by rendering the other side less so. At a community level, the same end is achieved by obtaining privileges for one's own party and enforcing discriminatory measures against and restrictions on the other. However, this traditional course is no longer universally followed. For example, in many parts of the world it is a long time since differences in religious outlook resulted in armed conflict. The still very acute clashes of interest between capital and labour are less and less tending to result in revolution. It may be that both parties to the conflict are becoming increasingly aware that to make the other party more insecure is no solution to the problem. It is now more usual to seek agreement on issues, and there is a growing appreciation that the good of one party may benefit the other. But though the likelihood of open conflict may be reduced, sufficient disagreement remains to keep both parties on the alert, which can be advantageous in itself.

It would be a direct application of mental health principles to situations of human conflict to introduce the notion that a greater degree of mutual security can be achieved only by making the other person more, and not less, secure. Our problem is to find ways in which to convince people that, ultimately, the key to the fulfilment of each lies in the safety and security of all. This view, far from being unrealistic, as often thought, faces and accepts the fact that differences in interest between groups can be very real and very significant. But they need not be mutually destructive; on the contrary, differences are capable of being turned to mutual advantage.

The attitude put forward here has a particularly poignant application to the example we have given of a minority group that is striving to maintain a privileged position in relation to the majority. The situation of the privileged minority is fraught with great anxiety, because of its fundamental insecurity. To maintain the attitude on which their position depends, the members of the minority group must block out from their minds all recognition of the inevitable long-term consequences of their attempt to undermine the security and to increase the inferiority feeling of the majority group. Such action can only greatly increase the dissatisfactions of the majority condemned to inferiority, and provoke greater retaliation in the long run. The tragic consequence of this type of solution when sought by a minority is that it cannot do otherwise than exacerbate the problem eventually, and make it insoluble on these terms.

Something analogous may be happening in connexion with the international arms race, which for a long time was restricted to a small and fairly homogeneous group of nations. Nowadays, both in armaments and in economic competition, this relatively small group of nations is attempting to maintain a privileged position in the face of the vast majority of less privileged people, and the latter are becoming increasingly aware of their relatively unfavourable situation. Consequently, the quality of anxiety and insecurity that arises among the members of the privileged group is becoming much more complicated and intense, because of the convergence of a number of new factors on the situation. Further, as remarked above, the recognition of the existence of a problem does not solve it, but may, in fact, increase the anxiety connected with it. The Study Group concluded that, where intergroup tension has arisen, the question of how one group may increase the feeling of security of the other, rather than undermine it, is one of the most vital for the future of the world.

These problems of intercommunication between different nations, or communities, or sections of a community, are much more complex, and acquire greater significance, when mutually incompatible ideologies are involved. One of the most difficult and perplexing tasks facing mental health action wherever it seeks to cross cultural or community boundaries is how to present aims and objectives in ways that are meaningful and acceptable in different cultures. Far too little thought has been given to the solution of the problems of communication of ideas between the various ideological blocs that have grown up, or between religious minorities and the other members of the communities in which the minority groups are living.

Mental health, in whatever culture, almost inevitably develops certain inherent values, and when cultural frontiers are crossed it may (and does) happen that these values become the target of a hostile ideological challenge. The resultant danger is one of stultification of further discussion and work in that particular area. The question is how can mental health action be presented in terms that do not invite an ideologically-based challenge and rejection.

In no areas of mental health work is opposition on ideological grounds more clearly manifest than in those that concern migration, population movements, and the setting up of new communities.

It appears to us to be of great urgency to find new and more acceptable ways of presenting this kind of issue to people in various countries, ways that secure sympathy and understanding and do not attract chauvinistic or xenophobic hostilities.

What we are looking for is not so much ideologically-free ideas and aims, as ways of describing areas of common interest in ideologically-free terms, so that all parties can get on with the task of exploring what needs to be done. The point can be illustrated by reference to the unprecedented growth of population in much of the world today, which is of concern to the whole world. In some circles this growth has been regarded as having sufficient dramatic urgency to earn the term 'population explosion'. As we shall note in Volume II, the individual may well regard a rapid population increase in his own country as a blessing, but a similar increase in a neighbouring country as a threat. The adoption in many places of the term 'population explosion' is a revelation of the anxiety that is felt about the world situation in this respect. However justified a feeling of anxiety may be, in view of our current incapacity to provide sufficient food even for the present total, it can only impair understanding of these matters if terms evocative of anxiety are attached to their discussion. We understand that the use of the term 'population explosion' has been criticized in the Soviet Union as an expression of venal Malthusianism, or, as stated more bluntly there, as the urgent wish of the capitalist world that the population of other countries shall not grow.

It is prudent in taking action on behalf of mental health to avoid the use of such terms, which, although they do not cause hostile feelings, being no more than an expression of a deeper underlying sentiment, tend to spread ambivalent attitudes. As noted above, massive population increases and population movements resulting from political and economic pressures have underlined the need, in very many countries, to find less emotionally biased modes of expressing attitudes to the stranger and the minority group in the community.

A semantic issue in regard to the term 'prejudice' is its current use virtually only for the negative or hostile aspects of stereotyping. Thus, prejudice is almost always 'against' something; but to find another term is far from easy. It has been suggested that 'prejudice' might be used to describe attitude, and 'discrimination' to describe forms of behaviour. Another solution is to use both 'prejudice' and 'discrimination' as strictly neutral terms, and to combine them with prepositions to express either a positive or a negative aspect. Thus, one can be prejudiced, or can discriminate, 'in favour of' or 'against'. In addition, 'to discriminate between' would indicate neutrality.

Neither of these terms can be regarded as wholly satisfactory by itself, primarily because of the attempt to compress too much special meaning into a word in common usage. Probably the best way to attach a lasting pejorative meaning to a concept that it is wished to oppose is by the use of an adjective like 'hostile', e.g. a hostile prejudice on the grounds of religion, race, culture, or whatever it may be.

In the case of prejudice, the over-simplification inherent in the use of a simple term to cover a complex field of individual or group relationships is the more significant because of the ambivalence that is a normal accompaniment of even violently hostile feelings. Strong hostility towards another individual or group is commonly accompanied by what might be termed almost a fascination, or even an infatuation, with the hated group; or at least by a preoccupation with the other party. Hostile prejudice is more than a matter of feelings of superiority and hostility; there is an accompanying deep ambivalence, which it is futile to attempt to combat by merely pointing out that the other party is not as bad as it is painted, that all human beings are equal, and so on. The ambivalence of the prejudiced person engenders defensive anxiety, and it can serve only to increase already existing anxiety to point out that feelings of superiority are rationally unfounded; as noted above in a related situation, to do so may heighten the current level of tension.

There is far more in these issues than the search for less evocative terms or the presentation of mental health concepts in ways that do not attract ideologically-based hostility. We are less concerned with the differences between people than with the positive contributions that each can make. In considering the future of mental health work, there is need to develop a programme of research and action with the aim of promoting a more positive sense of personal, family, and national identity. The focus of inquiry should be on the factors that contribute to a group's sense of distinctive identity, on the basis of its own qualities and achievements, and not on a basis of comparison with and derogation of the qualities of other groups. This point is related to the matter that we have already discussed of groups maintaining their sense of security and identity by virtue of their own qualities and without having recourse to causing insecurity among other groups. These issues will be taken up more fully in Volume II.

CHANGING EMPHASES IN MENTAL HEALTH WORK

As pointed out by Krapf and Moser (5), one of the most notable changes of emphasis in mental health work has been due to a wider realization of the need to reach a larger proportion of the population.

The movement to extend mental health provisions beyond the restricted aims of custodial care and segregation of the ill has nowhere in the world made an effective contribution over a period of longer than the last thirty years, and in much of the world even today has not made its mark. Attempts to reintegrate the insane into society – which have occurred sporadically in some countries over the centuries – have only in the last decade or so become of major significance.

Among the many factors contributing to the simultaneous emergence in a number of countries of a more liberal attitude towards the treatment of psychotics seems to have been the realization that problems of psychosis in the community can never be solved by therapeutic measures alone. Also, widespread increases in the population in general, and in the proportion of old people, have added to the overcrowding of hospital facilities, thus creating a situation of urgency for the community services

(92–99). A third factor has been the use of modern psychosocial and somatic therapies, and of psychotropic drugs, which has in some countries transferred the treatment of active psychotic illness from the hospital to the home and to the community at large.

In some parts of the world where, traditionally, the mentally sick have not been segregated in hospitals, ways are being sought to combine the benefits of retaining the mentally ill in the community with those of more modern therapeutic methods (75). It has sometimes been found that these modern approaches have been foreshadowed to some extent by traditional practices (228).

Modern therapy will be discussed more fully in Volume III, but it will be noted here that wherever active modern treatment of psychotic illness is undertaken in the community, there is a tendency for the whole concept of hospital bed provision for that community to be overhauled. A number of modern psychiatric inventions such as day hospitals, night hospitals, five-day-week hospitals, therapeutic social clubs, and so on, could have important applications also to the general hospital world.

As well as vast changes in hospital-based therapy, the spate of legislation in the mental health field in a number of countries is striking evidence of changing public attitudes. In some countries the alteration in the laws relating to the mentally ill and mentally defective reflects a virtual revolution in the minds of ordinary people.

Finally, in this connexion, the activities of mental health societies are multiplying all over the world. The response to World Mental Health Year has shown that many more organizations are doing useful things in the mental health field, in countries that had not previously been involved. This activity must presumably reflect a greater degree of community involvement.

GOVERNMENTAL ACTION IN THE FIELD OF MENTAL HEALTH

There has been so much recent governmental activity in the field of mental health that only a few examples can be referred to here. Governmental action can be seen at its highest potential in the work of the United Nations specialized agencies, and notably of the mental health units at the headquarters and regional offices of the World Health Organization; these latter have made an important impact on leaders in public health and cooperating disciplines throughout the world. Significant contributions have been made by WHO expert committees, working parties, and study groups, by a great number of consultant activities and by travelling fellowships; and by cooperative activities with individual governments and non-governmental organizations. UNESCO is not so explicitly concerned with mental health, but it has sponsored a number of important projects dealing with current moral and social problems: for example, those on international tensions, living in the world community, and, more specifically, mental health in education. UNESCO cooperated with Dr Margaret Mead acting on behalf of WFMH in the production of *Cultural Patterns and Technical Change* (504), which has sold 300,000 copies and been of immense help in the field of technical assistance. UNESCO also, on the suggestion of WFMH, published a collection of essays dealing with refugees, edited by Dr H. B. M. Murphy under the title *Flight and Resettlement* (542).

The UN Social Commission has shown an increasing interest in the provision of social workers and services, and has been associated with WFMH in a series of panel discussions on mental health and cultural change, problems of urbanization, and social and mental health changes in Africa. The International Labour Office has given increasing attention to the subject of human relations in industry; and the Food and Agriculture Organization to the mental health implications of nutrition problems. WFMH convened an interdisciplinary and inter-agency meeting to consider malnutrition and food habits, which resulted in a valuable publication in 1962 (483). A recent resurgence of interest in student mental health has led to conferences in several places.

These examples illustrate some of the recent happenings in governmental and intergovernmental action. Perhaps more significant is a growing realization that there are implications for mental health in the whole process of exchange in international meetings, that communication at this level needs very serious study to make it, at best, more effective or, at least, less dangerous. The contribution of mental health understanding to the conduct of international negotiations has not yet been explicit. A good deal has been written and thought about psychological factors in small group communication, and we would draw attention to WFMH's own publication (52). But in the WFMH meetings and UN assemblies, little more than a common-sense type of mental health approach has yet been attempted. However, even commonplace mental health contributions may have some therapeutic effect. For example, it is well recognized that aggression of one party towards another will provoke either counter-aggression or submission, rather than promote agreement. On the other hand, a firm but unaggressive resistance to an aggressive opening leaves possible a fresh start.

Another point, out of many that might be considered, is that of semantic difficulties. A word, a phrase, or a whole concept may mean different things to different people, although the same terms are being used. The subtler misunderstandings between two nationalities that share the same mother tongue may be no less difficult than the more obvious misunderstandings that occur between individuals conversing through an interpreter. Common sense suggests that it is always worth while in cases of obvious misunderstanding and conflict to go carefully over the ground and discover whether the parties are disputing about the same thing.

This whole concept of the place of mental health in government action is complex and difficult. The illustrations that have been given of intergovernmental action through the UN agencies have reflected the activities of individuals representing their own national governments, but working in an intergovernmental atmosphere. The attitudes which such people bring to their work are derived from their experiences in their own countries, but may be increasingly modified by mixing with representatives of other national governments in the common task. One specific difficulty in the development of both intergovernmental and non-governmental international action for mental health is that it is rarely possible for people to work in the international atmosphere and still retain a professional, and particularly a clinical, base at home. So that there is a tendency to develop a new and distinct class of international civil servant or professional employee of international non-governmental organizations which, in respect of the professional people engaged in the field of mental health, may mean an increasing separation between the individual worker and his professional base. This could be a source of weakness to the individual, who may be hampered in his own professional evolution.

Not the least of the dangers or difficulties affecting mental health work in governmental and intergovernmental action are those of getting involved in political situations, and the likelihood of their occurrence may be increased by the practice of facile interpretation of international situations in terms of small group and individual psychology, and especially of stereotyping. Mental health is concerned with principle and with the long-term view, and not with immediate political implications.

MULTIPLE INVOLVEMENT IN INTERNATIONAL WORK

It is insufficiently recognized that many different kinds of individuals are involved in mental health work and that, as we have remarked elsewhere, there are no such entities as mental health disciplines. All those who are professionally engaged in mental health work have a prior attachment to some more basic science or discipline. But whether a certain project is under the auspices of 'mental health', or psychiatry, sociology, or anthropology may be determined by chance, because of the small number of people available for employment, who, drawn from a variety of disciplines, will work in different locations under different auspices and in various combinations as opportunities arise.

We have referred above to the UNESCO manual on *Cultural Patterns and Technical Change* (504). This project was originally planned by the United States Committee on Food Habits in 1945, when Margaret Mead was the Executive Secretary and

Lawrence K. Frank the Chairman. A number of members of this Committee supported the foundation of the World Federation for Mental Health in 1948, and two years later the project was adopted by the WFMH Executive Board and recommended to UNESCO for support. It happened that the relevant head of department in UNESCO was a social psychologist who had been connected both with the US Committee on Food Habits and with the World Federation for Mental Health. In the event, the anthropologist who had been the Executive Chairman of the US Committee and who, in 1950, was a member of the WFMH Interprofessional Advisory Committee, was commissioned to undertake the preparation of the manual on behalf of the World Federation for Mental Health and financed by UNESCO. Thus the complex lines of communication in the mental health field resulted in this instance in a publication jointly to the credit of WFMH and UNESCO; but there are at least three or four different auspices under which, by another chain of circumstances, the same individuals could have undertaken the same job.

As we have remarked above (p. 90), it is very natural that people should demand to know precisely what the results of so-called mental health work may be, and our example illustrates how difficult it would be to assess exactly what resulted from which aspects of this mental health activity, or what resulted from the work of the same people under auspices other than those of mental health. To give another example: an official of a voluntary organization might draw the attention of a key official in the appropriate UN agency to the desirability of paying special attention to personal contacts between management and labour, and it may happen that this policy of improving human relations is followed with success in a number of countries. The general impression may develop that factory morale has improved, yet how is it possible to evaluate such 'results' and what proportion of the credit could be ascribed to the voluntary agency whose representative had acted as a catalyst?

It may appear futile to attempt to enumerate tangible results, and in mental health circles the view is gaining ground that the major objective should be not so much to achieve concrete and detailed effects in situations conceived to be disadvantageous as, instead, to create a changed climate of opinion in favour of increased activity by many different kinds of people in the interests of mental health. For example, it can hardly be possible ever to show to what extent mental health activity has been responsible for babies being fostered rather than brought up in institutions; or for hospitals showing more psychological insight in their maternity provisions; or for mediation and arbitration being preferred to aggression and conflict; or for intercultural conflicts being increasingly resolved on a basis of mutual understanding of cultural differences. In regard to the last point, in recent years it is noticeable how relevant publications by UN agencies and the like have dealt with cultural differences in a more sophisticated manner. Can this and other changes be ascribed to WFMH? It may well be claimed that the Federation has made a contribution, but it must be conceded that almost everyone in the psychological, sociological, and anthropological fields who is concerned with international questions has had some hand in bringing about the change of climate, whether, as is often the case, in connexion with the Federation, or under different and quite separate auspices.

It is even more difficult to find ways of evaluating mental health work precisely in relation to its objectives, because not only is the work often hampered by difficulties concerning its cultural application but also there may be a lack of clarity about the objectives themselves. Thus, although principles have been worked out for introducing new work in different areas, too often the new methods employed in practice have little relation to the culture. In the resulting failure the principles themselves have been increasingly condemned or rejected, and the real value of the mental health activity quite falsely judged.

The Study Group concluded that, for many years at least, it would not be possible to bring sufficient evidence of proof of achievement in mental health work to carry wide conviction. The effort is too polymorphic, too diffuse, and involves too many people working simultaneously under continuously changing auspices; so that to attempt to bring proof that 'mental health' achieved this or that would be not only downright misleading, but harmful, in that it would introduce competition and head-counting in a field in which cooperativeness is the most important consideration.

The difficulty in making an appraisal increases rather than decreases the importance of defining aims and objectives, in order to combat the insidious danger that relative inaccessibility to criticism on account of the absence of defined objectives may result in a certain diffuseness and irresponsibility of aim. On the other hand, criticism and suspicion may be aroused by the very vagueness of an organization's activities, as perceived by ordinary people in the community.

It can hardly be denied that the aims of mental health action are, in general, unclear, even in such a basic respect as whether it is primarily concerned with health or with an attempt to manipulate attitudes, albeit with the best of motives. We have referred above (p. 74) to a disquieting spirit of opposition that is sometimes expressed in accusations of brainwashing in the most pejorative sense of that term; or to the effect that 'mental health' is concerned not only with health but with influencing the feelings and loyalties of citizens in political directions conceived as wrong or subversive by the critics. In a less specific way, the question may often be asked, what right has an organization like the World Federation, with its national associates, to concern itself with public issues?

Although WFMH need not be too dismayed by such criticisms, it is very pertinent to inquire into the validity of the aspiration to operate at a level which requires the application of insights gained from the study of human relations to problems of public concern. Perhaps the Federation needs first to meet criticism from much nearer at hand, that its primary duty is with the international aspects of the management of the mentally ill, which responsibility is not adequately discharged at the present time. We have advocated above (p. 65) a concern with a favourable climate of opinion rather than exclusive attention to the righting of wrongs, and we question whether the wider responsibilities of mental health work can be divorced from the narrower aim of helping the mentally ill. In these two fields alone there would appear to be ample work that is within our current competence to keep us occupied for quite a long time.

PART THREE

Bibliography

Bibliography

This bibliography has been compiled with the primary aim of including a significant proportion of the more important and representative publications that have appeared since 1948 in the very wide field of mental health, as well as such other works as have been referred to in the text.

In so vast a field there is necessarily, and fortunately, considerable overlap between subjects and disciplines, which has led to the adoption of a somewhat arbitrary method of classification, for purposes of presentation.

Each section of the bibliography is divided into two parts:

(i) Works identified by individual authors. Here items are arranged alphabetically under authors' names. Works by the same author are given in chronological order, and where there are two or more works by the same author in the same year these are listed alphabetically according to the first letter of the title.

(ii) Works of collective authorship. These publications (reports, studies, etc.) are listed alphabetically under the name of the organization concerned, the title of the work, or the country of origin, as may be appropriate. Where it is necessary, items are given in chronological order or alphabetically by title, as in (i) above.

Abbreviations of titles of periodicals are, in general, those of the *World List of Scientific Periodicals* (3rd edition, London, 1952).

In psychiatry and allied disciplines, the following periodical reviews of the literature will be found to be the most useful:

Monthly – *Excerpta medica, Amsterdam*, Section VIII (Neurology and Psychiatry).

Annual – *Progress in Neurology and Psychiatry*, Ed. E. A. Spiegel, New York.

Annual – *Year Book of Neurology, Psychiatry and Neurosurgery*, Present Eds. R. P. Mackay, S. B. Wortis & O. Sugar, Chicago.

In other branches of the human sciences concerned, reference should be made to the respective specialized periodicals and year-books which periodically review the literature in these fields.

CLASSIFICATION

606 Psychiatry and the General Practitioner
609 Other Professional Training in the Mental Health Field
621 Audio-visual Aids

Public Education in Mental Health

630 Programmes and their Evaluation
636 Programmes for Parents
642 Popular Concepts of Mental Health
646 Use of the Mass Media

Additional References

Supplementary Titles

Unnumbered; a selection of more recent works

The Field of Mental Health

MENTAL HEALTH PLANNING AND PERSPECTIVES

1 BROCKINGTON, F. (ed.) 1955. *Mental Health and the World Community*. WFMH, London.

2 DUBOS, R. 1959. *Mirage of Health: Utopias, Progress and Biological Change*. London.

3 KRAPF, E. E. 1959. 'The international approach to the problems of mental health.' *Int. soc. Sci. J.* **11**: 63–71.

4 KRAPF, E. E. 1960. 'The work of the World Health Organization in the field of mental health.' *Ment. Hyg.* **44**: 315–338.

5 KRAPF, E. E. & MOSER, J. 1962. 'Changes of emphasis and accomplishments in mental health work, 1948–1960.' *Ment. Hyg.* **46**: 163–91. (Revised version of a working paper prepared for the Int. Study Group, Roffey Park, June 1961.)

6 LAIGNEL-LAVASTINE, M. & VINCHON, J. 1930. *Les Malades de l'esprit et leurs médecins du XVIe au XIXe siècle*. Paris. P. 14.

7 LEWIS, A. 1958. 'Between guesswork and certainty in psychiatry.' *Lancet* **1**: 171–5, 227–30.

8 PATON, A. C. L. & KIDSON, M. C. (eds.) 1961. *First World Mental Health Year: A Record*. WFMH, London.

9 REES, J. R. 1958. 'The way ahead.' *Amer. J. Psychiat.* **115**: 481–90.

10 SEMELAIGNE, R. 1930. *Les Pionniers de la psychiatrie française*. Tome 1. Paris.

11 THORNTON, E. M. (ed.) 1961. *Planning and Action for Mental Health* (12th & 13th Annual Meetings of WFMH – Barcelona, 1959 & Edinburgh, 1960). WFMH, London.

12 INTERNATIONAL PREPARATORY COMMISSION. 1948. *Mental Health and World Citizenship: A Statement prepared for the International Congress on Mental Health,*

London, 1948. WFMH, London. (English and German texts.)

13 WFMH. 1948. *Third International Congress on Mental Health, London, 1948.* Vol. 1: *History, Development and Organization*; Vol. 2: *Child Psychiatry*; Vol. 3: *Medical Psychotherapy*; Vol. 4: *Mental Hygiene.* 4 vols. WFMH, London.

14 WFMH. 1952. *Proceedings of the Fourth International Congress on Mental Health, Mexico City, 1951.* Mexico, D.F.

15 WFMH. 1954. *Mental Health in Public Affairs: A Report of the Fifth International Congress on Mental Health, Toronto, 1954.* Toronto.

16 WFMH. 1955. *Family Mental Health and the State* (8th Ann. Meeting WFMH, Istanbul, 1955). WFMH, London.

17 WFMH. 1956. *Bericht über die 6. Jahresversammlung der Weltvereinigung für Psychische Hygiene* (6th Ann. Meeting WFMH, Wien, 1953). Wien & Bonn.

18 WFMH. 1956. *Mental Health in Home and School* (9th Ann. Meeting WFMH, Berlin, 1956). WFMH, London.

19 WFMH. 1957. *Growing Up in a Changing World* (10th Ann. Meeting WFMH, Copenhagen, 1957). WFMH, London.

20 WFMH. 1960. *A Brief Record of Eleven Years, 1948–1959, and World Mental Health Year 1960.* WFMH, London.

21 WFMH. 1961. *Mental Health in International Perspective: A Review made in 1961 by an International and Interprofessional Study Group.* WFMH, London.

22 WFMH. 1961. *Proceedings of the VIth International Congress on Mental Health (Paris, 1961). Excerpta med. Int. Congr. Ser.* No. 45. Amsterdam.

23 WHO. 1950. Expert Committee on Mental Health: Report on the 1st Session. *World Hlth Org. tech. Rep. Ser.* 9. Geneva.

24 WHO. 1951. Expert Committee on Mental Health: Report on the 2nd Session. *World Hlth Org. tech. Rep. Ser.* 31. Geneva.

The Conceptualization of Mental Health

25 COBB, S. 1952. Foreword in *The Biology of Mental Health and Disease*. New York. Pp. xix–xxi.

26 DAVID, H. R. & BRENGELMANN, J. F. (eds.) 1960. *Perspectives in Personality Research*. London.

27 DICKS, H. V. 1959. *Mental Health in the light of Ancient Wisdom*. WFMH, London.

28 EL MAHI, T. 1960. 'Concept of mental health.' *E. Afr. med. J.* **37**: 472–6.

29 ERIKSON, E. H. 1956. 'The problem of ego identity.' *J. Amer. psychoanal. Ass.* **4**: 56–121.

30 GALDSTON, I. (ed.) 1960. *Human Nutrition, Historic and Scientific*. New York.

31 JAHODA, M. 1958. *Current Concepts of Positive Mental Health*. New York.

32 JUNG, C. G. 1958. *The Undiscovered Self* (transl. R. F. C. Hull). London.

33 KRAPF, E. E. 1961. 'The concepts of normality and mental health in psychoanalysis.' *Int. J. Psycho-Anal.* **42**: 439–46.

34 MASSERMAN, J. H. (ed.) 1959. *Individual and Familial Dynamics* (*Science and Psychoanalysis*, Vol. 2). New York. Part II: Familial and Social Dynamics. Pp. 90–214.

35 MASSERMAN, J. H. (ed.) 1960. *Psychoanalysis and Human Values* (*Science and Psychoanalysis*, Vol. 3). New York. Pp. 181–200.

36 MEAD, M. 1959. 'Mental health in world perspective.' In *Culture and Mental Health*, ed. M. K. Opler. New York. Pp. 501–16.

37 MEAD, M. 1962. 'Mental health and the wider world.' *Amer. J. Orthopsychiat.* **32**: 1–4.

38 RÜMKE, H. C. 1954. 'Solved and unsolved problems in mental health.' In *Mental Health in Public Affairs: A Report of the Fifth International Congress on Mental Health, Toronto*. Pp. 157 et seq.

39 SODDY, K. 1950. 'Mental health.' *Int. Hlth Bull. League of Red Cross Societies*, No. 2.

40 SODDY, K. (ed.) 1961. 'Identity.' In *Cross-cultural Studies in Mental Health*. London. Pp. 1–53.
(First published as: *WFMH Introductory Study No. 1*, London, 1957.)

41 SODDY, K. (ed.) 1961. 'Mental health and value systems.' In *Cross-cultural Studies in Mental Health*. London. Pp. 55–261.

42 WHEELIS, A. 1958. *The Quest for Identity*. New York.

43 MILBANK MEMORIAL FUND. 1952. *The Biology of Mental Health and Disease* (27th Ann. Conf. Milbank Memorial Fund). New York.

44 PIUS XII. 1960. *Pie XII parle de santé mentale et de psychologie*. Bruxelles.

Mental Health and Religion

45 ANDERSON, G. C. 1956. 'Psychiatry's influence on religion.' *Pastoral Psychology*, Sept.

46 ANDERSON, G. C. 1960. *Current Conditions and Trends in Relations between Religion and Mental Health*. New York.

47 APPEL, K. E. *et al.* 1959. 'Religion.' In *American Handbook of Psychiatry*, ed. S. Arieti. New York. Vol. 2: 1777–810.

48 OATES, W. E. 1955. *Religious Factors in Mental Illness*. New York.

49 O'DOHERTY, E. F. 1956. 'Religion and mental health.' *Studies*, Spring. Dublin.

50 TILLICH, P. J. 1960. *The Impact of Psychotherapy on Theological Thought*. New York.
(Also published in *Pastoral Psychology*, Feb. 1960.)

51 ACADEMY OF RELIGION AND MENTAL HEALTH. 1961. *Religion, Culture, and Mental Health* (Proc. 3rd Academy Symposium, Nov. 1959). New York.

Problems of Communication

52 CAPES, M. & WILSON, A. T. M. (eds.) 1960. *Communication or Conflict – Conferences: Their Nature, Dynamics, and Planning*. London.

53 CUNNINGHAM, J. M. 1952. 'Problems of communication in scientific and professional disciplines.' *Amer. J. Orthopsychiat.* **22**: 445–56.

54 EY, H. 1954. *Etudes psychiatriques.* Paris. Vol. 3: 32–45 (La Classification des maladies mentales).

55 FREMONT-SMITH, F. 1961. 'The interdisciplinary conference.' *Bull. Amer. Inst. biol. Sciences* **11**, No. 11 (Apr.): 17–20 & 32.

56 GLENN, E. S. 1954. 'Semantic difficulties in international communication.' *ETC: A Review of general Semantics* **11**: 163–80.

57 GLENN, E. S. *et al.* 1958. In *ETC: A Review of general Semantics* **15**: 81–151. Special issue on interpretation and intercultural communication (No. 2, Winter 1957–58).

58 RUESCH, J. 1958. 'Communication difficulties among psychiatrists.' In *Integrative Studies* (*Science and Psychoanalysis*, Vol. 1), ed. J. H. Masserman. New York. Pp. 85–100.

59 STENGEL, E. 1959. 'Classification of mental disorders.' *Bull. World Hlth. Org.* **21**: 601–63.

REGIONAL QUESTIONS

60 ARIETI, S. (ed.) 1959. *American Handbook of Psychiatry*. 2 vols. New York.

61 BARTON, W. E. *et al.* 1961. *Impressions of European Psychiatry*. Amer. Psychiatr. Ass., Washington, D.C.

62 BELLAK, L. 1961. *Contemporary European Psychiatry*. New York.

63 CARAVEDO, B. 1959. 'Social psychiatry in Peru.' In *Progress in Psychotherapy*, eds. J. H. Masserman & J. L. Moreno. New York. Vol. 4: 321.

64 CASEY, J. F. & RACKOW, L. L. 1960. *Observations on the Treatment of the Mentally Ill in Europe*. Veterans Admin., Washington, D.C.

65 CHU, L. & LIU, M. 1960. 'Mental diseases in Peking between 1933 and 1943.' *J. ment. Sci.* **106**: 274–80.

66 DAVIES, S. P. 1960. *Toward Community Mental Health: A Review of the First Five Years of Operations under the Community Mental Health Services Act of the State of New York*. New York.

67 DUCHÊNE, H. 1959. *Les Services psychiatriques publics extra-hospitaliers* (Rapport au 57e Congrès de Psychiatrie et de Neurologie de langue française, Tours, 1959). Paris.

68 FIELD, M. G. 1960. 'Approaches to mental illness in Soviet society: some comparisons and conjectures.' *Social Problems* 7: 277–97.

69 FORSTER, E. F. B. 1962. 'The theory and practice of psychiatry in Ghana.' *Amer. J. Psychother.* **16**: 7–51.

70 KLINE, N. S. 1960. *The Organization of Psychiatric Care and Psychiatric Research in the Union of Soviet Socialist Republics*. New York.

71 KRAPF, E. E. 1959. 'Les troubles mentaux des Africains et les problèmes de la psychiatrie comparée.' *Méd. et Hyg., Genève*, **17**: 123–30.

72 LAMBO, T. A. 1955. 'The role of cultural factors in paranoid psychosis among the Yoruba tribe (Nigeria).' *J. ment. Sci.* **101**: 239–66.

73 LAMBO, T. A. 1956. 'Neuropsychiatric observations in the Western Region of Nigeria.' *Brit. med. J.* **2**: 1388–94.

74 LAMBO, T. A. 1959. 'Mental health in Nigeria.' *World ment. Hlth.* **11**: 131–8. (Reprinted, ibid., 1961, **13**: 135–41.)

75 LAMBO, T. A. 1960. 'Further neuropsychiatric observations in Nigeria, with comments on the need for epidemiological study in Africa.' *Brit. med. J.* **2**: 1696–704.

76 LAMBO, T. A. 1960. 'The concept and practice of mental health in African cultures.' *E. Afr. med. J.* **37**: 464–71.

77 MARGETTS, E. L. 1960. 'The future for psychiatry in East Africa.' *E. Afr. med. J.* **37**: 448–56.

78 MORA, G. 1959. 'Recent American psychiatric developments.' In *American Handbook of Psychiatry*, ed. S. Arieti. New York. Vol. 1: 20–21.

79 PACHECO E SILVA, A. C. 1960. 'Mental hygiene in underdeveloped countries.' *World ment. Hlth* **12**: 18–23.

80 PATERSON, A. S. 1959. 'The practice of psychiatry in England under the National Health Service, 1948–1959.' *Amer. J. Psychiat.* **116**: 244–50.

81 SIVADON, P. 1958. 'Problèmes de santé mentale en Afrique noire.' *World ment. Hlth* **10**: 106–19.

82 SIVADON, P. 1959. 'Problèmes de santé mentale aux Caraïbes.' *World ment. Hlth* **11**: 122–30.

83 STOLLER, A. 1957. 'An Australian looks at the underdeveloped world.' In *Mental Health and the World Community*, ed. F. Brockington. WFMH, London. Pp. 31–9.

84 STRÖMGREN, E. 1958. 'Mental health service planning in Denmark.' *Danish med. Bull.* **5**: 1–17.

85 TOOTH, G. 1950. *Studies in Mental Illness in the Gold Coast.* Colonial Res. Publ. No. 6. Colonial Office, London.

86 VYNCKE, J. 1957. 'Psychoses et nèvroses en Afrique centrale.' *Mém. Acad. R. Sci. colon.* Bruxelles, N.S., 5: fasc. 5.

87 WORTIS, J. 1961. 'A psychiatric study tour of the USSR.' *J. ment. Sci.* **107**: 119–56.

88 CCTA/CSA. 1960. *Mental Disorders and Mental Health in Africa South of the Sahara (Bukavu, 1958)*. Publ. No. 35. London.

89 *East African med. J.*, 1960. **37**: 443–85 (No. 6, June). Special Number: World Mental Health Year, 1960.

90 'The social problem of epilepsy in Peru.' 1960. *Amer. J. Psychiat.* **117**: 163–4.

91 WHO. 1959. *Seminar on Mental Health in Africa South of the Sahara (Brazzaville, 1958): Final Report.* WHO Regional Office for Africa, Brazzaville.

LOCAL PROGRAMMES

92 CARSE, J., PANTON, N. E. & WATT, A. 1958. 'A district mental health service: The Worthing experiment.' *Lancet* **1**: 39–41.

93 COLEMAN, M. D. & ZWERLING, I. 1959. 'The psychiatric emergency clinic: A flexible way of meeting mental health needs.' *Amer. J. Psychiat.* **115**: 980–4.

94 FREEMAN, H. L. 1960. 'Oldham and District psychiatric service.' *Lancet* **1**: 218–21.

95 LEMKAU, P. V. & CROCETTI, G. M. 1961. 'The Amsterdam municipal psychiatric service: A psychiatric-sociological review.' *Amer. J. Psychiat.* **117**: 779–83.

96 LEYBERG, J. T. 1959. 'A district psychiatric service: The Bolton pattern.' *Lancet* **2**: 282–4.

97 LIN, T. 1961. 'Evolution of mental health programmes in Taiwan.' *Amer. J. Psychiat.* **117**: 961–71.

98 QUERIDO, A. 1954. 'Domiciliary psychiatry: The Amsterdam experiment.' *Brit. med. J.* **2**: 1043.

99 QUERIDO, A. 1956. 'Early diagnosis and treatment services.' In *The Elements of a Community Mental Health Program.* Milbank Memorial Fund, New York. Pp. 158–181.

CLINICAL ASPECTS OF MENTAL HEALTH ACTION

100 EDINBURGH CORPORATION. 1959. *Mental Health Services – Edinburgh: A Plan for Co-ordinated Development*. Report by a Medical Working Party. Edinburgh.

101 NEW YORK STATE. 1954. *New Program for Community Mental Health Services*. Dept. of Mental Hygiene, Albany, N.Y.

102 WHO. 1959. Conference on Mental Hygiene Practice (Helsinki, 1959). Report of Committee B: Community Psychiatric Services. WHO Regional Office for Europe, Copenhagen. (Duplicated document.)

SURVEYS AND EPIDEMIOLOGICAL STUDIES

103 BLACKER, C. P. 1946. *Neurosis and the Mental Health Services*. London.

104 FELIX, R. H. & KRAMER, M. 1953. 'Extent of the problem of mental disorders.' *Ann. Amer. Acad. polit. soc. Sci.* 1953: 5–14.

105 FREMMING, K. H. 1947. *Morbid Risk of Mental Diseases in an Average Danish Population*. Copenhagen, (Also published as: *The Expectation of Mental Infirmity in a Sample of a Danish Population*, London, 1951.)

106 HALLGREN, B. & SJÖGREN, T. 1959. 'A clinical and genetico-statistical study of schizophrenia and low-grade mental deficiency in a large Swedish rural population.' *Acta psychiat.* **35**, *Suppl.* 140. Copenhagen.

107 HOCH, P. H. & ZUBIN, J. (eds.) 1961. *Comparative Epidemiology of the Mental Disorders* (Proc. 49th Ann. Meeting Amer. Psychopathol. Ass., 1959). New York.

108 HUGHES, C. C. *et al.* 1960. *People of Cove and Woodlot* (*The Stirling County Study of Psychiatric Disorder and Sociocultural Environment*, Vol. 2). New York.

109 JACO, E. G. 1960. *The Social Epidemiology of Mental Disorders: A Psychiatric Survey of Texas*. New York.

110 KRAMER, M. 1953. 'Long-range studies of mental hospital patients, an important area for research in chronic disease.' *Milbank mem. Fund Quart.* **31**: 253–64.

111 KRAMER, M. 1957. 'A discussion of the concepts of incidence and prevalence as related to epidemiologic studies of mental disorders.' *Amer. J. publ. Hlth* **47**: 826–40.

112 LEIGHTON, A. H. 1959. *My Name is Legion* (*The Stirling County Study of Psychiatric Disorder and Sociocultural Environment*, Vol. 1). New York.

113 MURPHY, J. M. 1962. 'Cross-cultural studies of the prevalence of psychiatric disorders.' *World ment. Hlth* **14**: 53–65.

114 NORRIS, V. 1959. *Mental Illness in London* (Maudsley Monogr. No. 6). London.

115 OPLER, M. K. 1958. 'Epidemiological studies of mental illness: methods and scope of the Midtown study in New York.' In *Symposium on Preventive and Social Psychiatry* (April 1957). Walter Reed Army Institute of Research, Washington, D.C. Pp. 111–47.

116 PASAMANICK, B. (ed.) 1959. *Epidemiology of Mental Disorder*. Amer. Ass. Advanc. Sci., Washington, D.C.

117 PASAMANICK, B. 1961. 'Survey of mental disease in urban population: IV. Approach to total prevalence rates.' *Arch. gen. Psychiatr.* **5**: 151–5.

118 PLUNKETT, R. J. & GORDON, J. E. 1960. *Epidemiology and Mental Illness*. New York.

119 PRIMROSE, E. J. R. 1962. *Psychological Illness: A Community Study*. (Re: General practice.) London.

120 REID, D. D. 1960. *Epidemiological Methods in the Study of Mental Disorders* (World Hlth Org. publ. Hlth Papers 2). Geneva.

121 RÜMKE, H. C. 1961. 'Identification of mental disorder and its causes.' In *Planning and Action for Mental Health*, ed. E. M. Thornton. WFMH, London. Pp. 222–8.

122 SHEPHERD, M. 1957. *A Study of the Major Psychoses in an English County* (Maudsley Monogr. No. 3). London.

123 SJÖGREN, T. & LARSSON, T. 1959. 'The changing age-structure in Sweden and its impact on mental illness.' *Bull. World Hlth. Org.* **21**: 569–82.

124 SROLE, L. *et al.* 1962. *Mental Health in the Metropolis* (Midtown Manhattan Study). New York.

125 ZUBIN, J. (ed.) 1961. *Field Studies in the Mental Disorders* (Proc. Work Conf., Amer. Psychopathol. Ass., 1959). New York.

126 GROUP FOR THE ADVANCEMENT OF PSYCHIATRY (GAP). 1961. *Problems of Estimating Changes in Frequency in Mental Disorders.* Report No. 50. New York.

127 JAPAN. 1959. Report of the statistical survey of the mentally disordered in 1954. Ministry of Health & Welfare, Tokyo. (Duplicated document.)

128 MILBANK MEMORIAL FUND. 1950. *Epidemiology of Mental Disorder.* New York.

129 WHO. 1960. Epidemiology of Mental Disorders: 8th Report of the Expert Committee on Mental Health. *World Hlth Org. tech. Rep. Ser.* 185. Geneva.

130 WHO. 1961. 'The epidemiology of mental disorders.' *World Hlth Org. Chron.* **15**: 68.

Clinical Action in the Community

131 AHRENFELDT, R. H. 1958. *Psychiatry in the British Army in the Second World War.* London & New York.

132 ibid. 'Practical Considerations on the Disposal of Delinquents in the Army.' Appendix A, pp. 264–8.

133 BIERER, J. 1960. 'Past, present and future.' *Int. J. soc. Psychiat.* **6**: 165–73.

134 BIERER, J. 1961. 'Day hospitals: further developments.' *Int. J. soc. Psychiat.* **7**: 148–51.

135 EHRHARDT, H. *et al.* (eds.) 1958. *Psychiatrie und Gesellschaft: Ergebnisse und Probleme der Sozialpsychiatrie.* Bern & Stuttgart.

136 FERGUSON, R. S. 1961. 'Side-effects of community care.' *Lancet* **1**: 931–2.

137 GINZBERG, E. *et al.* 1959. *The Ineffective Soldier: Lessons for Management and the Nation.* Vol. 1: *The Lost Divisions*;

Vol. 2: *Breakdown and Recovery*; Vol. 3: *Patterns of Performance*. 3 vols. New York.

138 GREENBLATT, M., LEVINSON, D. J. & KLERMAN, G. J. 1961. *Mental Patients in Transition*. Springfield, Ill.

139 HORDER, J. 1961. The Role of Public Health Officers and General Practitioners in Mental Health Care (Working Paper No. 1, May 1961). WHO Expert Committee on Mental Health, Geneva, Oct.–Nov. 1961. (Duplicated document.)

140 JONES, M. 1961. 'Intra and extramural community psychiatry.' *Amer. J. Psychiat.* **117**: 748–7.

141 JONES, M. & RAPOPORT, R. N. 1955. 'Administrative and social psychiatry.' *Lancet* **2**: 386–8.

142 LEIGHTON, A. H., CLAUSEN, J. A. & WILSON, R. N. (eds.) 1957. *Explorations in Social Psychiatry*. New York.

143 MACMILLAN, D. 1958. 'Community treatment of mental illness.' *Lancet* **2**: 201–4.

144 MACMILLAN, D. 1961. 'Community mental health services and the mental hospital.' *World ment. Hlth* **13**: 46–58.

145 MAY, A. R. 1961. 'Prescribing community care for the mentally ill.' *Lancet* **1**: 760–1.

146 MCKERRACHER, D. G. 1961. 'Psychiatric care in transition.' *Ment. Hyg.* **45**: 3–9.

147 REES, T. P. 1957. 'Back to moral treatment and community care.' *J. ment. Sci.* **103**: 303–13.

148 ROLLIN, H. R. 1960. 'Social psychiatry in Britain.' *Trans. Coll. Physicians Philad. Ser.* 4, **27**: 126–37.

149 TITMUSS, R. M. 1961. As reported in *Lancet* **1**: 609.

150 VEIL, C. 1959. 'Introduction à la psychiatrie sociale.' *Bull. Centre Etudes Rech. psychotech.* **8**: 29–38.

151 'Doubtful progress in psychiatry' (Correspondence). 1960. *Lancet* **2**: 261, 371, 433, 599–600.

152 ENGLAND & WALES. 1951. *Report of the Committee on Social Workers in the Mental Health Services*. Ministry of Health, London.

153 WHO. 1954. *European Seminar on Mental Health Aspects of*

Public Health Practice (Amsterdam, 1953). WHO Regional Office for Europe, Geneva.

154 WHO. 1955. 'Mental health through public health practice.' *World Hlth Org. Chron.* **9**: 247–53.

155 WHO. 1959. Social Psychiatry and Community Attitudes: 7th Report of the Expert Committee on Mental Health. *World Hlth Org. tech. Rep. Ser.* 177. Geneva.

THE PSYCHIATRIC HOSPITAL

I. *Changing Patterns of Organization*

156 BAKER, A. A. 1958. 'Breaking up the mental hospital.' *Lancet* **2**: 253–5.

157 BAKER, A. A., DAVIES, R. L. & SIVADON, P. 1959. *Psychiatric Services and Architecture.* (World Hlth Org. publ. Hlth Papers 1). Geneva.

158 BARR, A., GOLDING, D. & PARNELL, R. W. 1962. 'Recent critical trends in mental hospital admissions in the Oxford Region.' *J. ment Sci.* **108**: 59–67.

159 BARTON, R., ELKES, A. & GLEN, F. 1961. 'Unrestricted visiting in a mental hospital: An inquiry into its effects and nursing-staff attitudes.' *Lancet* **1**: 1220–2.

160 BATEMAN, J. F. 1949. In *Better Care in Mental Hospitals* (Proc. 1st Mental Hospital Institute, Amer. Psychiat. Ass.). Washington, D.C. Appendix III, p. 187.

161 BERESFORD, C. 1959. Annual Report of The Retreat mental hospital, York, for 1959 – as quoted in *Lancet* **2**: 680.

162 BRIDGMAN, R. F. 1955. *The Rural Hospital: Its Structure and Organization* (World Hlth Org. Monogr. Ser. 21). Geneva.

163 CLARK, D. H. 1958. 'Administrative therapy: Its clinical importance in the mental hospital.' *Lancet* **1**: 805–8.

164 COOPER, A. B. & EARLY, D. F. 1961. 'Evolution in the mental hospital: Review of a hospital population.' *Brit. med. J.* **1**: 1600–3.

165 FLECK, S. *et al.* 1957. 'Interaction between hospital staff and families.' *Psychiatry* **20**: 343–50.

166 GARRATT, F. N., LOWE, C. R. & MCKEOWN, T. 1958. 'Institutional care of the mentally ill.' *Lancet* **1**: 682–4.

167 GREENBLATT, M. *et al.* 1955. *From Custodial to Therapeutic Patient Care in Mental Hospitals.* New York. (Cf. 'Relation of the hospital to the community.' Pp. 212–34.)

168 HARPER, J. 1959. 'Out-patient adult psychiatric clinics.' *Brit. med. J.* **1**: 357–60.

169 JONES, K. & SIDEBOTHAM, R. 1962. *Mental Hospitals at Work.* London.

170 KINGSTON, F. E. 1962. 'Trends in mental-hospital population and their effect on planning.' *Lancet* **2**: 49.

171 LINDSAY, J. S. B. 1962. 'Trends in mental-hospital population and their effect on planning.' *Lancet* **1**: 1354–5.

172 MACMILLAN, D. 1958. 'Hospital-community relationships.' In *An Approach to the Prevention of Disability from Chronic Psychoses: The Open Mental Hospital within the Community.* Milbank Memorial Fund, New York. Pp. 29–50.

173 MAIN, T. F. 1958. 'Mothers with children in a psychiatric hospital.' *Lancet* **2**: 845–7.

174 NORTON, A. 1961. 'Mental hospital ins and outs: A survey of patients admitted to a mental hospital in the past 30 years.' *Brit. med. J.* **1**: 528–36.

175 OVERHOLSER, W. 1955. 'The present status of the problems of release of patients from mental hospitals.' *Psychiat. Quart.* **29**: 372–80.

176 REPOND, A. 1960. 'Santé mentale et hôpital psychiatrique.' *Rev. Méd. prév.* **5**: 276–98.

177 RICHTER, D. (ed.) 1950. *Perspectives in Neuropsychiatry.* London.

178 SANDS, S. L. 1959. 'Discharges from mental hospitals.' *Amer. J. Psychiat.* **115**: 748–50.

179 SHAW, D. & SAMUEL, A. 1959. 'Medical administration in psychiatric hospitals.' *Lancet* **2**: 170–2.

180 SIVADON, P. 1959. 'Transformation d'un service d'aliénés

de type classique en un centre de traitement actif et de réadaptation sociale.' *Bull. World Hlth Org.* **21**: 593–600.

181 SMITH, S. *et al.* 1960. 'Metamorphosis of a mental hospital.' *Lancet* **2**: 592–3.

182 TOOTH, G. C. 1958. 'The psychiatric hospital and its place in a mental health service.' *Bull. World Hlth Org.* **19**: 363–87.

183 TOOTH, G. C. & BROOKE, E.M. 1961. 'Trends in the mental hospital population and their effect on future planning.' *Lancet* **1**: 710–13.

184 'A different hospital.' 1959. *Lancet* **2**: 221–2.

185 'A look at mental hospitals.' 1962. *Lancet* **1**: 900.

186 ENGLAND & WALES. 1962. *A Hospital Plan for England and Wales.* London.
(Preface and general review reprinted verbatim in *Brit. med. J.* 1962, **1**: 244–51.)

187 'Gains in outpatient psychiatric services, 1959.' 1960. *Publ. Hlth Rep.* 75: 1092–4. Washington, D.C.

188 'Hospital services for the mentally ill.' 1961. *Brit. med. J.* **1**: 1184.

II. *The Therapeutic Community*

189 CAUDILL, W. 1958. *The Psychiatric Hospital as a Small Society.* Cambridge, Mass.

190 CROCKET, R. W. 1960. 'Doctors, administrators, and therapeutic communities.' *Lancet* **2**: 359–63.

191 JONES, M. *et al.* 1952. *Social Psychiatry: A Study of Therapeutic Communities.* London.

192 MAIN, T. F. 1946. 'The hospital as a therapeutic institution.' *Bull. Menninger Clin.* **10**: 66–70.

193 STANTON, A. H. & SCHWARTZ, M. S. 1954. *The Mental Hospital: A Study of Institutional Participation in Psychiatric Illness and Treatment.* New York.

194 WALTER REED ARMY INSTITUTE OF RESEARCH. 1958. 'Panel on the development of a therapeutic milieu in the mental hospital.' In *Symposium on Preventive and Social Psychiatry (April 1957).* Washington, D.C. Pp. 455–529.

195 WHO. 1953. Expert Committee on Mental Health: 3rd Report. *World Hlth Org. tech. Rep. Ser.* 73. Geneva.

III. *Day and Night Hospitals*

196 BIERER, J. 1951. *The Day Hospital: An Experiment in Social Psychiatry and Syntho-Analytic Psychotherapy*. London.

197 BIERER, J. 1959. 'Theory and practice of psychiatric day hospitals.' *Lancet* **2**: 901–2.

198 BIERER, J. & BROWNE, I. W. 1960. 'An experiment with a psychiatric night hospital.' *Proc. R. Soc. Med.* **53**: 930–2.

199 BOAG, T. J. 1960. 'Further developments in the day hospital.' *Amer. J. Psychiat.* **116**: 801–6.

200 CAMERON, D. E. 1956. 'The day hospital.' In *The Practice of Psychiatry in General Hospitals* by A. E. Bennett *et al.* Berkeley & Los Angeles, Calif. Pp. 134–50.

201 CRAFT, M. 1959. 'Psychiatric day hospitals.' *Amer. J. Psychiat.* **116**: 251–4.

202 FARNDALE, J. 1961. *The Day Hospital Movement in Great Britain*. Oxford.

203 FOX, R. *et al.* 1960. 'Psychiatric day hospitals.' *Lancet* **1**: 824–5.

204 FREEMAN, H. L. 1960. 'The day hospital.' *World ment. Hlth* **12**: 192–8.

205 GOSHEN, G. E. 1959. 'New concepts of psychiatric care with special reference to the day hospital.' *Amer. J. Psychiat.* **115**: 808–11.

IV. *Rehabilitation*

206 BRIDGER, H. 1946. 'The Northfield experiment.' *Bull. Menninger Clin.* **10**: 71–6.

207 GRAYSON, M. *et al.* 1952. *Psychiatric Aspects of Rehabilitation*. New York Univ., Bellevue Med. Center, New York.

208 GREENBLATT, M. & SIMON, B. (eds.) 1959. *Rehabilitation of the Mentally Ill*. Amer. Ass. Advanc. Sci., Washington, D.C.

209 LE GUILLANT, L. *et al.* 1958. 'Une réforme de l'assistance psychiatrique: Le service médico-social de secteur.' *Tech. hosp.* **14**: 34.

210 WHO. 1958. Expert Committee on Medical Rehabilitation: 1st Report. *World Hlth Org. tech. Rep. Ser.* 158. Geneva.

PSYCHOTHERAPY

211 FERENCZI, S. 1955. *Final Contributions to the Problems and Methods of Psycho-Analysis* (ed. M. Balint). London. P. 141.

212 FROMM-REICHMANN, F. & MORENO, J. L. (eds.) (Vol. 1); MASSERMAN, J. H. & MORENO, J. L. (eds.) (Vols. 2–5). 1956–60. *Progress in Psychotherapy*. 5 vols. New York.

213 MASSERMAN, J. H. & MORENO, J. L. (eds.) 1959. *Progress in Psychotherapy*, Vol 4: *Social Psychotherapy*. New York.

PHARMACOTHERAPY

214 BRILL, H. & PATTON, R. E. 1959. 'Analysis of population reduction in New York State mental hospitals during the first four years of large scale therapy with psychotropic drugs.' *Amer. J. Psychiat.* **116**: 495–509.

215 GARATTINI, S. & GHETTI, V. (eds.) 1957. *Psychotropic Drugs* (Proc. Int. Symposium on Psychotropic Drugs, Milan 1957). Amsterdam.

216 GELBER, I. 1959. *Release Mental Patients on Tranquillizing Drugs and the Public Health Nurse*. New York.

217 GROSS, M. 1960. 'The impact of ataractic drugs on a mental hospital out-patient clinic.' *Amer. J. Psychiat.* **117**, 444–7.

218 GUPTA, J. C., DEB, A. K. & KAHALI, B. S. 1943. 'Preliminary observations on the use of *Rauwolfia serpentina Benth.* in the treatment of mental disorders.' *Indian med. Gaz.* **78**: 547–9.

219 HOCH, P. H. 1959. 'Drug therapy.' In *American Handbook of Psychiatry*, ed. S. Arieti. New York. Vol. 2: 1541–51.

220 HUTCHINSON, J. T. & SMEDBERG, D. 1960. 'Phenelzine ("Nardil") in the treatment of endogenous depression.' *J. ment. Sci.* **106**: 704–10.

221 HUTCHINSON, R. 1953. 'Modern treatment.' *Brit. med J.* **1**: 671.

222 JACOBSEN, E. 1959. 'The comparative pharmacology of some psychotropic drugs.' *Bull. World Hlth Org.* **21**: 411–93.

223 KILOH, L. G. & BALL, J. R. B. 1961. 'Depression treated with imipramine ("Tofranil"): A follow-up study.' *Brit. med. J.* **1**: 168–71.

224 KLINE, N. S. 1959. 'Psychopharmaceuticals: Effects and side-effects.' *Bull. World Hlth Org.* **21**: 397–410.

225 KLINE, N. S. (ed.) 1959. *Psychopharmacology Frontiers* (2nd Int. Congr. Psychiatry: Proc. Psychopharmacol. Symposium). Boston.

226 LINDEMANN, E. 1959. 'The relation of drug-induced mental changes to psychoanalytical theory.' *Bull. World Hlth Org.* **21**: 517–26.

227 LINN, E. L. 1959. 'Sources of uncertainty in studies of drugs affecting mood, mentation or activity.' *Amer. J. Psychiat.* **116**: 97–103.

228 PRINCE, R. 1960. 'The use of *Rauwolfia* for the treatment of psychoses by Nigerian native doctors.' *Amer. J. Psychiat.* **117**: 147–9.

229 REES, L., BROWN, A. C. & BENAIM, S. 1961. 'A controlled trial of imipramine ("Tofranil") in the treatment of severe depressive states.' *J. ment. Sci.* **107**: 552–9.

230 REES, L. & DAVIES, B. 1961. 'A controlled trial of phenelzine ("Nardil") in the treatment of severe depressive illness.' *J. ment. Sci.* **107**: 560–6.

231 SANDISON, R. A. 1959. 'The role of psychotropic drugs in group therapy.' *Bull. World Hlth Org.* **21**: 505–15.

232 SANDISON, R. A. 1959. 'The role of psychotropic drugs in individual therapy.' *Bull. World Hlth Org.* **21**: 495–503.

233 UHR, L. & MILLER, J. G. (eds.) 1960. *Drugs and Behavior.* New York.

234 WATT, J. M. & BREYER-BRANDWIJK, M. G. 1962. *The Medicinal and Poisonous Plants of Southern and Eastern Africa.* (2nd ed.) Edinburgh. Pp. 95–100.

235 PIUS XII. 1960. 'Psychiatrie et psychopharmacologie (1958).' In *Pie XII parle de santé mentale et de psychologie.* Bruxelles. Pp. 72–75 (and cf. E. E. Krapf, Préface, p. 10).

236 WHO. 1958. Ataractic and Hallucinogenic Drugs in Psychiatry; Report of a Study Group. *World Hlth Org. tech. Rep. Ser.* 152. Geneva.

PSYCHIATRY IN THE GENERAL HOSPITAL

237 BENNETT, E. A. *et al.* 1956. *The Practice of Psychiatry in General Hospitals.* Berkeley & Los Angeles, Calif.

238 BENNETT, A. E. 1959. 'Problems in establishing and maintaining psychiatric units in general hospitals.' *Amer. J. Psychiat.* **115**: 974–9.

239 BROOK, C. P. B. & STAFFORD-CLARK, D. 1961. 'Psychiatric treatment in general wards.' *Lancet* **1**: 1159–62.

240 COHEN, N. A. & HALDANE, F. P. 1962. 'Inpatient psychiatry in general hospitals.' *Lancet* **1**: 1113–14.

241 COTTON, J. M. 1961. 'The function of a psychiatric service in a general hospital.' *Mental Hosp.*, Sept., pp. 4–7.

242 HOENIG, J. & CROTTY, I. M. 1959. 'Psychiatric inpatients in general hospitals.' *Lancet* **2**: 122–3.

243 LINN, L. 1955. *A Handbook of Hospital Psychiatry: A Practical Guide to Therapy.* New York.

244 LINN, L. (ed.) 1961. *Frontiers in General Hospital Psychiatry.* New York.

245 MOROSS, H. 1954. 'The administration of a psychiatric service in a general hospital.' *S. Afr. med. J.* **28**: 886–9.

246 NOBLE, H. N. 1961. As reported in *Brit. med. J.* **1**: 664–5.

247 SMITH, S. 1961. 'Psychiatry in general hospitals: Manchester's integrated scheme.' *Lancet* **1**: 1158–9.

248 'Psychiatry in the general hospital.' 1962. *Lancet* **1**: 1107.

Psychiatry in Obstetric Practice

249 HARGREAVES, G. R. 1955. 'Obstetrics and psychiatry.' *Lancet* **1**: 39–40.

250 MORRIS, N. 1960. 'Human relations in obstetric practice.' *Lancet* **1**: 913–15.

251 ENGLAND & WALES. 1961. *Human Relations in Obstetrics.* Ministry of Health, London.

Psychiatry in General Practice

252 BALINT, M. 1957. *The Doctor, his Patient and the Illness.* London.

253 FRANKLIN, L. M. 1960. 'An appraisal of psychiatry in general practice.' *Brit. med. J.* **2**: 451–3.

254 KRAPF, E. E. 1956. 'Tâches et possibilités du médecin de famille dans le domaine de l'hygiène mentale.' *Arch. suisses Neurol. Psychiat.* 77: 47–56.
(English transl.: 'The family doctor's tasks and opportunities in the field of mental hygiene.' *J. Amer. med. Women's Ass.*, 1957, **12**: 212-15.)

255 LEMERE, F. & KRAABEL, A. B. 1959. 'The general practitioner and the psychiatrist.' *Amer. J. Psychiat.* **116**: 518–521.

256 WATTS, C. A. H. 1958. 'Management of chronic psychoneurosis in general practice.' *Lancet* **2**: 362–4.

257 COLLEGE OF GENERAL PRACTITIONERS. 1958. 'Psychological medicine in general practice.' *Brit. med. J.* **2**: 585–90.

The Mental Health of the General Hospital

258 BARNES, E. 1959. 'Mental health in general hospitals.' *World ment. Hlth* **11**: 43–7.

259 BARNES, E. 1961. *People in Hospital.* London.

260 BLUESTONE, E. M. 1958. 'Fear in hospital practice: Some advantages of home care.' *Lancet* **1**: 1083–4.

261 HEASMAN, G. A. 1962. 'The patient, the doctor and the hospital.' *Lancet* **2**: 59–62.

262 STATHAM, C. 1959. 'Noise and the patient in hospital: A personal investigation.' *Brit. med. J.* **2**: 1247–8.

263 ENGLAND & WALES. 1953. *The Reception and Welfare of In-Patients in Hospitals.* Ministry of Health, London.

264 ENGLAND & WALES. 1961. *The Pattern of the In-Patient's Day.* Ministry of Health, London.

265 KING EDWARD'S HOSPITAL FUND FOR LONDON. 1958. *Noise Control in Hospitals.* London.
(Cf. *Lancet*, 1958, **2**: 1269.)

266 KING EDWARD'S HOSPITAL FUND FOR LONDON. 1962. *Information Booklets for Patients.* London.
(Cf. *Lancet*, 1962, **1**: 1392–3.)

267 SCOTTISH ASS. MENTAL HEALTH. 1960. *Report of Scottish Study Group on Psychological Problems in General Hospitals.* Edinburgh.

THE MENTAL HEALTH OF CHILDREN

I. *Clinical Problems*

268 BRADLEY, C. 1941. *Schizophrenia in Childhood.* New York. Pp. 21–4.

269 BROCK, J. F. & AUTRET, M. 1952. *Kwashiorkor in Africa* (World Hlth Org. Monogr. Ser. 8). Geneva.

270 FREEDMAN, A. M. 1959. 'Day hospitals for severely schizophrenic children.' *Amer. J. Psychiat.* **115**: 893–8.

271 GEBER, M. & DEAN, R. F. A. 1955. 'Psychological factors in the aetiology of kwashiorkor.' *Bull. World Hlth Org.* **12**: 471–5.

272 JELLIFFE, D. B. 1955. *Infant Nutrition in the Subtropics and Tropics* (World Hlth Org. Monogr. Ser. 29). Geneva.

273 KANNER, L. 1959. 'Trends in child psychiatry.' *J. ment. Sci.* **105**: 581–93.

274 LORAND, S. & SCHNEER, H. I. (eds.) 1961. *Adolescents: Psychoanalytic Approach to Problems and Therapy.* New York.

275 LURIA, A. K. 1961. *The Role of Speech in the Regulation of Normal and Abnormal Behaviour* (ed. J. Tizard). Oxford.

276 MOSSE, H. L. 1958. 'The misuse of the diagnosis, childhood schizophrenia.' *Amer. J. Psychiat.* **114**: 791–4.

277 SHAGASS, C. & PASAMANICK, B. (eds.) 1960. *Child Development and Child Psychiatry.* In Tribute to Dr Arnold Gesell in his Eightieth Year. Washington, D.C.

278 SODDY, K. 1960. *Clinical Child Psychiatry.* London.

279 TANNER, J. M. & INHELDER, B. (eds.) 1956–60. *Discussions on Child Development.* 4 vols. London.

280 TIZARD, J. P. M. *et al.* 1959. 'The role of the paediatrician in mental illness.' *Lancet* **2**: 193–5.

281 AMERICAN PSYCHIATRIC ASSOCIATION. 1957. *Psychiatric Inpatient Treatment of Children.* Washington, D.C.

282 CENTRE INTERNATIONAL DE L'ENFANCE. 1953. *Les Problèmes de l'enfance dans les pays tropicaux de l'Afrique* (Brazzaville, 1952). Paris. Pp. 315–61.

II. *Organization of Services*

283 BUCKLE, D. & LEBOVICI, S. 1960. *Child Guidance Centres* (World Hlth Org. Monogr. Ser. 40). Geneva.

284 CONNELL, P. H. 1961. 'The day hospital approach in child psychiatry.' *J. ment. Sci.* **107**: 969–77.

285 CREAK, M. 1959. 'Child health and child psychiatry: neighbours or colleagues?' *Lancet* **1**: 481–5.

286 POLLAK, O. *et al.* 1952. *Social Science and Psychotherapy for Children.* New York.

287 SMALLPEICE, V. 1958. 'Children as day patients.' *Lancet* **2**: 1366–7.

288 ENGLAND & WALES. 1955. *Report of the Committee on Maladjusted Children.* Ministry of Education, London.

289 WHO. 1952. *Scandinavian Seminar on Child Psychiatry and Child Guidance Work* (Lillehammer, 1952). WHO Regional Office for Europe, Geneva.

290 WHO. 1952. Joint Expert Committee on the Physically Handicapped Child: 1st Report. *World Hlth Org. tech. Rep. Ser.* 58. Geneva.

III. *Children in Hospital*

291 CAPES, M. 1955. 'The child in hospital.' *Bull. World Hlth Org.* **12**: 427–70.

292 ILLINGWORTH, R. S. 1958. 'Children in hospital.' *Lancet* **2**: 165–71.

293 TREADGOLD, S. 1960. 'Billy goes to hospital.' *Med. biol. Illustr.* **10**: 191–6.

294 BRITISH PAEDIATRIC ASS. 1959. 'The welfare of children in hospital.' *Brit. med. J.* **1**: 166–9.

295 ENGLAND & WALES. 1959. *The Welfare of Children in Hospital.* Ministry of Health, London.

Some Specific Areas of Mental Health Concern

I. *Addiction*

296 DUHL, L. J. 1959. 'Alcoholism: The public health approach – A new look from the viewpoint of human ecology.' *Quart. J. Stud. Alc.* **20**: 112–25.

297 JELLINEK, E. M. 1960. *The Disease Concept of Alcoholism.* New Haven.

298 JELLINEK, E. M. *et al.* 1955. 'The "craving" for alcohol: A symposium by members of the WHO Expert Committees on Mental Health and on Alcohol.' *Quart J. Stud. Alc.* **16**: 34–66.

299 KILOH, L. G. & BRANDON, S. 1962. 'Habituation and addiction to amphetamines.' *Brit. med. J.* **2**: 40–3.

300 KRUSE, H. D. (ed.) 1961. *Alcoholism as a Medical Problem.* New York.

301 CALIFORNIA. 1961. *Reports of the Division of Alcoholic Rehabilitation of the Department of Public Health (State of California).* Publ. No. 1: A Study of Community Concepts and Definitions (Pt. I); Publ. No. 2: Selected Aspects of the Prospective Follow-up Study (a preliminary review); Publ. No. 3: Criminal Offenders and Drinking Involvement (a preliminary analysis).

302 WHO. 1951. *European Seminar and Lecture Course on Alcoholism* (Copenhagen, 1951). WHO Regional Office for Europe, Geneva.

303 WHO. 1951–55. Expert Committee on Mental Health – Alcoholism Sub-committee: 1st and 2nd Reports; Expert Committee on Alcohol: 1st Report; Alcohol and Alcoholism: Report of an Expert Committee. *World Hlth Org. tech. Rep. Ser.* 42, 48, 84, 94. Geneva.

304 WHO. 1955. *European Seminar on the Prevention and Treatment of Alcoholism*: Selected Lectures (Noordwijk, 1954). WHO Regional Office for Europe, Geneva. (Reprinted from *Quart. J. Stud. Alc.* 1954, **15**, and 1955, **16**.)

305 WHO. 1957–61. Treatment and Care of Drug Addicts: Report of a Study Group; Expert Committee on Addiction-Producing Drugs: 10th and 11th Reports. *World Hlth Org. tech. Rep. Ser.* 131, 188, 211. Geneva.

II. *Ageing*

306 ANDERSON, J. E. (ed.) 1956. *Psychological Aspects of Aging.* Amer. Psychol. Ass., Washington, D.C.

307 BASH, K. W. 1959. 'Mental health problems of aging and the aged from the viewpoint of analytical psychology.' *Bull. World Hlth Org.* **21**: 563–8.

308 COSIN, L. Z. 1955. 'The place of the day hospital in the geriatric unit.' *Int. J. soc. Psychiat.* **1**: No. 2, 33–41.

309 HARGREAVES, G. R. *et al.* 1962. 'Psychiatric and geriatric beds' (Central Consultants and Specialists Committee). As reported in *Brit. med. J., Suppl.* **1**: 209–10.

310 HOCH, P. H. & ZUBIN, J. (eds.) 1961. *Psychopathology of Aging* (Proc. 50th Ann. Meeting Amer. Psychopathol. Ass., 1960). New York.

311 ROTH, M. 1959. 'Mental health problems of aging and the aged.' *Bull. World Hlth Org.* **21**: 527–61, 563–91.

312 SHELDON, J. H. 1960. 'Problems of an ageing population.' *Brit. med. J.* **1**: 1223–30.

313 WHO. 1959. Mental Health Problems of Aging and the Aged: 6th Report of the Expert Committee on Mental Health. *World Hlth Org. tech. Rep. Ser.* 171. Geneva.

III. *Cyclothymia*

314 GIBSON, R. W. *et al.* 1959. 'On the dynamics of the manic-depressive personality.' *Amer. J. Psychiat.* **115**: 1101–7.

315 STENSTEDT, A. 1959. 'Involutional melancholia: An etiologic, clinical and social study of endogenous depression in later life, with special reference to genetic factors.' *Acta psychiat.* **34**, *Suppl.* 127, Copenhagen.

IV. *Delinquency and Criminality*

316 BOVET, L. 1951. *Psychiatric Aspects of Juvenile Delinquency* (World Hlth Org. Monogr. Ser. 1). Geneva.

317 EDELSTON, H. 1952. *The Earliest Stages of Delinquency: A Clinical Study from the Child Guidance Clinic.* Edinburgh.

318 GIBBENS, T. C. N. 1961. *Trends in Juvenile Delinquency* (World Hlth Org. publ. Hlth Papers 5). Geneva.

319 GITTINS, J. 1952. *Approved School Boys: An Account of the Observation, Classification and Treatment of Boys who come to Aycliffe School.* Home Office, London. (Cf. esp. Pt. III, pp. 84 ff., on psychiatric and psychometric investigations.)

320 JONES, H. 1960. *Reluctant Rebels: Re-education and Group Process in a Residential Community.* London.

321 MANNHEIM, H. & WILKINS, L. T. 1955. *Prediction Methods in Relation to Borstal Training.* London.

V. *Migration*

322 EITINGER, L. 1960. 'The symptomatology of mental disease among refugees in Norway.' *J. ment. Sci.* **106**: 947–66.

323 LISTWAN, I. A. 1959. 'Mental disorders in migrants: Further study.' *Med. J. Australia*, April. (Reprinted in *World ment. Hlth*, 1960, **12**: 38–45.)

324 MEZEY, A. G. 1960. 'Personal background, emigration and mental disorder in Hungarian refugees.' *J. ment. Sci.* **106**: 618–27.

325 MEZEY, A. G. 1960. 'Psychiatric aspects of human migrations.' *Int. J. soc. Psychiat.* **5**: 245–60.

326 MEZEY, A. G. 1960. 'Psychiatric illness in Hungarian refugees.' *J. ment Sci.* **106**: 628–37.

VI. *Neurosis, and Physical and Psychosomatic Illness*

327 BARKER, R. G. *et al.* 1953. *Adjustment to Physical Handicap and Illness: A Survey of the Social Psychology of Physique and Disability.* Social Sci. Res. Council, New York.

328 BARTON, R. 1959. *Institutional Neurosis.* Bristol.

329 CLECKLEY, H. M. 1959. 'Psychopathic states.' In *American Handbook of Psychiatry*, ed. S. Arieti. New York. Vol. 1: 567–88.

330 COHEN OF BIRKENHEAD, LORD. 1958. 'Epilepsy as a social problem.' *Brit. med. J.* **1**: 672–5.

331 DERNER, G. F. 1953. *Aspects of the Psychology of the Tuberculous.* New York.

332 KRAPF, E. E. 1957. 'On the pathogenesis of epileptic and hysterical seizures.' *Bull. World Hlth Org.* **16**: 749–62.

333 LJUNGBERG, L. 1957. 'Hysteria: A clinical, prognostic and genetic study.' *Acta psychiat.* **32**, *Suppl.* 112. Copenhagen.

334 LOWINGER, P. 1959. 'Leprosy and psychosis.' *Amer. J. Psychiat.* **116**: 32–7.

335 MANSON-BAHR, P. E. C. 1960. 'The physical background of mental disorder in Africans.' *E. Afr. med. J.* **37**: 477–9.

336 MARS, L. 1955. *La Crise de possession: Essais de psychiatrie comparée.* Port-au-Prince, Haiti.

337 MILLER, H. 1961. 'Accident neurosis.' *Brit. med. J.* **1**: 919–25, 992–8.

338 TANNER, J. M. (ed.) 1960. *Stress and Psychiatric Disorder* (2nd. Oxford Conf. Ment. Health Res. Fund). Oxford.

339 WITTKOWER, E. D. 1955. *A Psychiatrist Looks at Tuberculosis.* (2nd ed.) London.

340 WITTKOWER, E. D. & CLEGHORN, R. A. (eds.) 1954. *Recent Developments in Psychosomatic Medicine*. London.

341 WITTKOWER, E. D. & RUSSELL, B. 1953. *Emotional Factors in Skin Disease*. New York.

342 YAP, P. M. 1960. 'The possession syndrome: A comparison of Hong Kong and French findings.' *J. ment. Sci.* **106**: 114–37.

343 ENGLAND & WALES. 1956. *Report of the Sub-committee on the Medical Care of Epileptics*. Ministry of Health, London.

344 PIUS XII. 1960. 'Ressources psycho-spirituelles dans la réhabilitation des malades de la lèpre (1956).' In *Pie XII parle de santé mentale et de psychologie*. Bruxelles. Pp. 68–9.

345 WHO. 1957. Juvenile Epilepsy: Report of a Study Group. *World Hlth Org. tech. Rep. Ser.* 130. Geneva.

346 WHO. 1961. 'Rehabilitation in leprosy.' *World Hlth Org. Chron.* **15**: 111.

VII. *Schizophrenia*

347 BROWN, G. W. 1960. 'Length of stay and schizophrenia: A review of statistical studies.' *Acta psychiat.* **35**: 414–30.

348 FLECK, S. 1960. 'Family dynamics and origin of schizophrenia.' *Psychosom. Med.* **22**: 333–44.

349 LIDZ, T. & FLECK, S. 1959. 'Schizophrenia, human integration, and the role of the family.' In *Etiology of Schizophrenia*, ed. D. Jackson. New York. Pp. 323–45.

350 LIDZ, T. *et al.* 1957. 'The intrafamilial environment of the schizophrenic patient: I. The father.' *Psychiatry* **20**: 329–42.

351 WING, J. K. 1960. 'Pilot experiment in the rehabilitation of long-hospitalized male schizophrenic patients.' *Brit. J. prev. soc. Med.* **14**: 173–80.

352 WING, J. K. & BROWN, G. W. 1961. 'Social treatment of chronic schizophrenia: A constructive survey of three mental hospitals.' *J. ment. Sci.* **107**: 847–61.

353 *Second International Congress for Psychiatry (Zürich)*. 1957. *Congress Report*. Zürich. Vol. 1 (contains a number of papers on schizophrenia in various cultures).

354 WHO. 1959. Report of World Health Organization Study Group on Schizophrenia – Geneva, 9–14 September 1959. *Amer. J. Psychiat.* **115**: 865–72.

VIII. *Subnormality*

355 ADAMS, M. (ed.) 1960. *The Mentally Subnormal: The Social Casework Approach*. London.

356 CLARKE, A. M. & CLARKE, A. D. B. (eds.) 1958. *Mental Deficiency: The Changing Outlook*. London.

357 CRAFT, M. 1959. 'Personality disorder and dullness.' *Lancet* **1**: 856–8.

358 EARL, C. J. C. 1961. *Subnormal Personalities: Their Clinical Investigation and Assessment*; with additional material by H. C. Gunzburg. London.

359 JERVIS, G. A. 1959. 'The mental deficiencies.' In *American Handbook of Psychiatry*, ed. S. Arieti. New York. Vol. 2: 1312–13.

360 LEWIS, A. J. 1960. 'The study of defect' (Adolf Meyer Research Lecture). *Amer. J. Psychiat.* **117**: 289–305.

361 O'GORMAN, G. 1958. 'A hospital for the psychotic-defective child.' *Lancet* **2**: 951–3.

362 SLAUGHTER, S. S. 1960. *The Mentally Retarded Child and his Parent*. New York.

363 TIZARD, J. 1953. 'The prevalence of mental subnormality.' *Bull. World Hlth Org.* **9**: 423–40.

364 TIZARD, J. & GRAD, J. C. 1961. *The Mentally Handicapped and their Families: A Social Survey* (Maudsley Monogr. No. 7). London.

365 TOKUHATA, G. K. & STEHMAN, V. A. 1961. 'Sociologic implications, and epidemiology, of mental disorders in recent Japan.' *Amer. J. publ. Hlth* **51**: 697–705.

366 WHO. 1954. The Mentally Subnormal Child. *World Hlth Org. tech. Rep. Ser.* 75. Geneva.

367 WHO. 1957. *European Seminar on the Mental Health of the Subnormal Child* (Oslo, 1957). WHO Regional Office for Europe, Copenhagen.

IX. *Suicide*

368 CAPSTICK, A. 1960. 'Urban and rural suicide.' *J. ment. Sci.* **106**: 1327–36.

369 SAINSBURY, P. 1955. *Suicide in London: An Ecological Study*. London.

370 STENGEL, E. 1960. 'The complexity of motivations to suicidal attempts.' *J. ment. Sci.* **106**: 1388–93.

371 VEIL, C. 1957. 'Note sur la gravité et l'urgence en psychiatrie de dispensaire.' *Ann. médico-psychol.* **2**: 124–7.

372 YAP, P. M. 1958. *Suicide in Hong Kong*. Hong Kong.

Preventive Aspects of Mental Health Action

PROMOTION OF MENTAL HEALTH IN THE COMMUNITY

373 CAPLAN, G. 1961. *An Approach to Community Mental Health.* London.

374 FRASER, F. 1958. 'Medical practice in a changing society.' *Lancet* **1**: 154–7.

375 GOTTLIEB, J. S. & HOWELL, R. W. 1957. 'The concepts of "prevention" and "creativity development" as applied to mental health.' In *Four Basic Aspects of Preventive Psychiatry*, ed. R. H. Ojemann. State Univ. Iowa, Iowa City. Pp. 9–17.

376 JONES, K. 1960. *Mental Health and Social Policy, 1845–1959.* London. (Cf. especially Chap. 11, 'Problems and Experiments, 1948–59'; pp. 153–77.)

377 KEBRIKOV, O. V. *et al.* 1954. *Reports of the Members of the Soviet Delegation at the Fifth Congress on Mental Health Defence.* Moscow.

378 KRAPF, E. E. 1955. 'Structure and functions of the Mental Health Society.' *Ment. Hyg.* **39**: 225–31.

379 KRAPF, E. E. 1958. 'The work of the World Health Organization in relation to the mental health problems in changing cultures.' In *Growing Up in a Changing World.* WFMH, London. Pp. 106–12.

380 KRUSE, H. D. (ed.) 1957. *Integrating the Approaches to Mental Disease.* (2 Conferences held under the auspices of the Committee of Public Health, N.Y. Acad. Med.) New York.

381 LEMKAU, P. V. 1952. 'Toward mental health: Areas that promise progress.' *Ment. Hyg.* **36**: 197–209.

382 MACMILLAN, D. 1960. 'Preventive geriatrics: Opportunities of a community mental health service.' *Lancet* **2**: 1439–41.

383 SIVADON, P. & DUCHÊNE, H. 1958. 'Santé mentale, hygiène mentale et prophylaxie mentale.' In *Traité de psychiatrie: Encyclopédie médico-chirurgicale*. Paris. Tome 3, art. 37960 A30, p. 3.

384 STEVENSON, G. S. 1956. *Mental Health Planning for Social Action*. New York.

385 TUFTS, E. M. 1955. 'The field of mental health promotion.' In *Community Programs for Mental Health*, ed. R. Kotinsky & H. L. Witmer. Cambridge, Mass. Pp. 33–45.

386 WILLIAMS, C. D. 1958. 'Social medicine in developing countries.' *Lancet* **1**: 863–6, 919–22.

387 *Constructive Mental Hygiene in the Caribbean* (Proc. 1st Caribbean Conf. on Mental Health, March 1957). Assen.

388 MILBANK MEMORIAL FUND. 1956. *The Elements of a Community Mental Health Program*. New York. Pp. 101–5 & 122–34.
(G. R. Hargreaves: The Protection of the Personality.)

389 UNITED STATES. 1961. Joint Commission on Mental Illness and Health, *Action for Mental Health*. New York. (Cf. Summary, 'Action for Mental Health: Digest of Final Report.' *Modern Hosp.*, 1961, **96**, 109–24.)

390 WHO. 1957. The Psychiatric Hospital as a Centre for Preventive Work in Mental Health: 5th Report of the Expert Committee on Mental Health. *World Hlth Org. tech. Rep. Ser.* 134. Geneva.

391 WHO. 1961. Programme Development in the Mental Health Field: 10th Report of the Expert Committee on Mental Health. *World Hlth Org. tech. Rep. Ser.* 223. Geneva.

Public Health in Action

392 GRUENBERG, E. M. 1957. 'Application of control methods to mental illness.' *Amer. J. publ. Hlth.* **47**: 944–52.

393 HARGREAVES, G. R. 1958. *Psychiatry and the Public Health*. London.

394 LEMKAU, P. V. 1955. *Mental Hygiene in Public Health*. (2nd ed.) New York. Pp. 11 et seq.

395 UNITED KINGDOM. 1956. *An Inquiry into Health Visiting: Report of a Working Party on the Field of Work, Training and Recruitment of Health Visitors.* Ministry of Health, Dept of Health for Scotland, and Ministry of Education, London.

LEGISLATION

396 DAVIDSON, H. A. 1959. 'The commitment procedures and their legal implications.' In *American Handbook of Psychiatry*, ed. S. Arieti. New York. Vol 2: 1902–22.

397 GOTTLIEB, J. S. & TOURNEY, G. 1958. 'Commitment procedures and the advancement of psychiatric knowledge.' *Amer. J. Psychiat.* **115**: 109–13.

398 GRAY, H. R. 1960. 'The reform of the law relating to mental health.' *New Zealand med. J.* **59**: 18–23.

399 MACLAY, W. S. 1960. 'The new Mental Health Act in England and Wales.' *Amer. J. Psychiat.* **116**: 777–81.

400 ENGLAND & WALES. 1948. *National Health Service Act, 1946: Provisions Relating to the Mental Health Services.* Ministry of Health, London.

401 SCOTLAND. 1955. *The Law Relating to Mental Illness and Mental Deficiency in Scotland: Proposals for Amendment.* Dept of Health, Edinburgh.

402 SCOTLAND. 1959. *Mental Health Legislation: 2nd Report by a Committee appointed by the Council.* Dept. of Health & Scottish Health Services Council, Edinburgh.

403 'The Mental Health Act.' 1960. *Brit. med. J.* **2**: 1297–8.

404 UNITED KINGDOM. 1957. *Royal Commission on the Law relating to Mental Illness and Mental Deficiency, 1954–1957: Report.* London.

405 WHO. 1955. *Hospitalization of Mental Patients: A Survey of Existing Legislation.* Geneva.

406 WHO. 1955. Legislation Affecting Psychiatric Treatment: 4th Report of the Expert Committee on Mental Health. *World Hlth Org. tech. Rep. Ser.* 98. Geneva.

Mental Health in Infancy

407 BOWLBY, J. 1951. *Maternal Care and Mental Health* (World Hlth Org. Monogr. Ser. 2). Geneva.

408 BOWLBY, J. 1958. 'Separation of mother and child.' *Lancet* **1**: 480.

409 BOWLBY, J. 1958. 'The nature of the child's tie to his mother.' *Int. J. Psycho-Anal.* **39**: 350–73.

410 FOSS, B. M. (ed.) 1961. *Determinants of Infant Behaviour: Proceedings of a Tavistock Study Group on Mother-Infant Interaction* (Ciba Foundation, Sept. 1959). London.

411 MEAD, M. 1954. 'Some theoretical considerations on the problem of mother-child separation.' *Amer. J. Orthopsychiat.* **24**: 471–83.

412 MURPHY, L. B. *et al.* 1956. *Personality in Young Children.* 2 vols. New York.

413 STONE, F. H. 1958. 'Early disorders of the mother-child relationship.' *Lancet* **1**: 1115–18.

414 'Problèmes d'hygiène mentale posés par la séparation des jeunes enfants de leur mère.' 1957. *Hyg. Ment.* No 1.

415 WHO. 1962. *Deprivation of Maternal Care: A Reassessment of its Effects* (World Hlth Org. publ. Hlth Papers 14). Geneva.

The Welfare of Children

416 BACKETT, E. M. & JOHNSTON, A. M. 1959. 'Social patterns of road accidents to children: Some characteristics of vulnerable families.' *Brit. med. J.* **1**: 409–13.

417 BAUCHARD, P. 1953. *The Child Audience: A Report on Press, Film and Radio for Children.* UNESCO, Paris.

418 CAPLAN, G. (ed.) 1961. *Prevention of Mental Disorder in Children: Initial Explorations.* London.

419 DUHRSSEN, A. 1958. *Heimkinder und Pflegekinder in ihrer Entwicklung.* Göttingen.

420 GINZBERG, E. (ed.) 1960. *The Nation's Children.* Vols 1 & 3. New York.

421 HIMMELWEIT, H. T. *et al.* 1958. *Television and the Child.* London.

422 HOCHFELD, E. & VALK, M. A. 1953. *Experience in Inter-Country Adoptions.* Int. Social Service (Amer. Branch), New York.

423 WERTHAM, F. 1954. *Seduction of the Innocent.* New York.

424 ENGLAND & WALES. 1955. *Seventh Report on the Work of the Children's Department: November 1955.* Home Office, London.

425 ENGLAND & WALES. 1960. *Report of the Committee on Children and Young Persons.* Home Office, London.

426 UNITED KINGDOM. 1954. *Report of the Departmental Committee on the Adoption of Children.* Home Office & Scottish Home Dept, London.

427 WHO. 1953. Joint UN/WHO Meeting of Experts on the Mental Health Aspects of Adoption: Final Report. *World Hlth Org. tech. Rep. Ser.* 70. Geneva.

428 WHO. 1957. Accidents in Childhood: Facts as a Basis for Prevention – Report of an Advisory Group. *World Hlth Org. tech. Rep. Ser.* 118. Geneva.

429 WHO. 1959. 'Accidents in childhood in the Americas.' *World Hlth Org. Chron.* **13**: 249–50.

430 WHO. 1960. *Seminar on the Prevention of Accidents in Childhood* (Spa, 1958). WHO Regional Office for Europe, Copenhagen.

The Family

431 ACKERMAN, N. W. *The Psychodynamics of Family Life.* New York.

432 BLACKER, C. P. 1958. 'Disruption of marriage: Some possibilities of prevention.' *Lancet* **1**: 578–81.

433 EISENSTEIN, V. W. (ed.) 1956. *Neurotic Interaction in Marriage.* New York.

434 LIN, T. (ed.) 1960. *Reality and Vision: A Report of the First Asian Seminar on Mental Health and Family Life* (Baguio, 1958). Manila.

MENTAL HEALTH AND THE EDUCATIONAL SYSTEM

435 ANDERSON, H. H. *et al.* 1959. 'Image of the teacher by adolescent children in four countries: Germany, England Mexico, United States.' *J. soc. Psychol.* **50**: 47–55.

436 BONNEY, M. E. 1960. *Mental Health in Education.* Boston.

437 BOWER, E. M. 1960. *Early Identification of Emotionally Handicapped Children in School.* Springfield, Ill.

438 KAPLAN, L. 1959. *Mental Health and Human Relations in Education.* New York.

439 KRUGMAN, M. (ed.) 1958. *Orthopsychiatry and the School.* New York.

440 MACFARLANE, J. W. 1953. 'The uses and predictive limitations of intelligence tests in infants and young children.' *Bull. World Hlth Org.* **9**: 409–15.

441 SHIPLEY, J. T. 1961. *The Mentally Disturbed Teacher.* Philadelphia.

442 WALL, W. D. 1955. *Education and Mental Health* (Problems in Education XI). UNESCO, Paris.

443 WHEELER, O., PHILLIPS, W. & SPILLANE, J. P. 1961. *Mental Health and Education.* London.

444 ENGLAND & WALES. 1952. *The Health of the School Child: Report of the Chief Medical Officer of the Ministry of Education for 1950 and 1951.* Ministry of Education, London.

445 SCOTTISH COUNCIL FOR RESEARCH IN EDUCATION. 1953. *Social Implications of the 1947 Scottish Mental Survey.*

446 SCOTTISH COUNCIL FOR RESEARCH IN EDUCATION. 1959. *Educational . . . Aspects of the 1947 Scottish Mental Survey.*

447 WHO. 1951. Expert Committee on School Health Services: Report on the 1st Session. *World Hlth Org. tech. Rep. Ser.* 30: pp. 14–16. Geneva.

STUDENT MENTAL HEALTH

448 BLAINE, G. & MACARTHUR, C. 1961. *Emotional Problems of the Student.* New York.

449 DAVIDSON, M. A. *et al.* 1955. 'The detection of psychological vulnerability in students.' *J. ment. Sci.* **101**: 810–25.

450 DAVY, B. W. 1960. 'The sources and prevention of mental ill-health in university students.' *Proc. R. Soc. Med.* **53**: 764–9.

451 FARNSWORTH, D. L. 1957. *Mental Health in College and University*. Cambridge, Mass.

452 FARNSWORTH, D. L. 1959. 'Social and emotional development of students in college and university.' *Ment. Hyg.* **43**: 358–67, 568–76.

453 FUNKENSTEIN, D. H. (ed.) 1959. *The Student and Mental Health: An International View* (Proc. 1st Int. Conf. Student Mental Health, Princeton, 1956). Cambridge, Mass.

454 FUNKENSTEIN, D. H. & WILKIE, G. H. 1956. *Student Mental Health: An annotated Bibliography, 1936–1955*. WFMH, London; Int. Ass. Universities, Paris.

455 PRINCE, R. 1960. 'The "brain fag" syndrome in Nigerian students.' *J. ment. Sci.* **106**: 559–70.

456 ROOK, A. 1959. 'Student suicides.' *Brit. med. J.* **1**: 599–603.

457 WAGGONER, R. W. & ZEIGLER, T. W. 1961. 'Psychiatric factors in medical students in difficulty: A follow-up study.' *Amer. J. Psychiat.* **117**: 727–31.

458 WEDGE, B. M. (ed.) 1958. *Psychosocial Problems of College Men*. Div. of Student Mental Hygiene, Yale Univ.; New Haven, Conn.

459 INT. ASS. UNIVERSITIES, 1958. *Student Mental Health* (Papers Int. Ass. Universities, No. 3). Paris.

Industrial Mental Health

460 KOEKEBAKKER, J. 1955. 'Mental Health and Group Tensions.' *Bull. World Hlth Org.* **13**: 543–50.

461 LING, T. M. (ed.) 1954. *Mental Health and Human Relations in Industry*. London.

462 LING, T. M. 1955. 'La santé mentale dans l'industrie.' *Bull. World Hlth Org.* **13**: 551–9.

463 MINDUS, E. 1955. 'Outlines of a concept of industrial psychiatry.' *Bull. World Hlth Org.* **13**: 561–74.

464 VEIL, C. 1957. 'Aspects médico-psychologiques de l'industrialisation moderne.' *Rev. int. Travail*, **75**. (English transl.: 'Medical and psychological aspects of modern industry.' *Int. Labour Rev.* **75**.)

465 VEIL, C. 1961. 'Hygiène mentale du travailleur.' In *Traité de psychiatrie: Encyclopédie médico-chirurgicale*. Paris. Tome 3, art. 37960 A50.

466 UNITED KINGDOM. 1958. *Final Report of the Joint Committee on Human Relations in Industry 1954–57; and Report of the Joint Committee on Individual Efficiency in Industry 1953–57*. Dept Sci. Indust. Res. & Med. Res. Council, London.

467 WFMH. 1948. *Third International Congress on Mental Health, London 1948*. Vol. 4: *Mental Hygiene*. London. Pp. 175–209 (Mental Health in Industry and Industrial Relations).

468 WHO. 1953. Joint ILO/WHO Committee on Occupational Health: 2nd Report. *World Hlth Org. tech. Rep. Ser.* 66. Geneva.

469 WHO. 1957. Joint ILO/WHO Committee on Occupational Health: 3rd Report. *World Hlth Org. tech. Rep. Ser.* 135. Geneva.

470 WHO. 1958. *Human Relations and Mental Health in Industrial Units*. WHO Regional Office for Europe, Copenhagen.

471 WHO. 1959. Mental Health Problems of Automation: Report of a Study Group. *World Hlth Org. tech. Rep. Ser.* 183. Geneva.

Prevention of Crime and Delinquency

472 GLUECK, S. & GLUECK, E. T. 1950. *Unraveling Juvenile Delinquency*. New York.

473 GLUECK, S. & GLUECK, E. T. 1959. *Predicting Delinquency and Crime*. Cambridge, Mass.

474 GUTTMACHER, M. S. 1949. 'Medical aspects of the causes and prevention of crime and the treatment of offenders.' *Bull. World Hlth Org.* **2**: 279–88.

475 GUTTMACHER, M. S. 1950. 'Psychiatric examination of offenders.' *Bull. World Hlth Org.* **2**: 743–9.

476 LECONTE, M. 1960. 'De la nécessité de tirer quelques enseignements de l'actualité de la criminalité psychiatrique révélée par la presse.' *Ann. Méd. lèg.* **40**: 246–63.

477 LOPEZ-REY, M. 1958. 'Mental health and the work of the United Nations in the field of the prevention of crime and the treatment of offenders.' In *Growing Up in a Changing World.* WFMH, London. Pp. 93–100.

478 ENGLAND & WALES. 1959. *Penal Practice in a Changing Society: Aspects of Future Development (England and Wales).* Home Office, London.

479 ENGLAND & WALES. 1960. *Criminal Law Revision Committee: 2nd Report (Suicide).* Home Office, London.

480 UN DEPT. OF SOCIAL AFFAIRS. 1953. *Int. Rev. crim. Policy.* Special issue on Medical, Psychological, and Social Examination of Offenders.

481 UN DEPT. OF SOCIAL AFFAIRS. 1959. European Consultative Group on the Prevention of Crime and Treatment of Offenders (4th Session, Geneva, 1958). *Int. Rev. crim. Policy* **14**: 59–69.

482 UNESCO. 1957. *The University Teaching of Social Sciences: Criminology.* Paris.

Social and Cross-cultural Aspects of Mental Health Action

Health and Human Welfare

483 BURGESS, A. & DEAN, R. F. A. (eds.) 1962. *Malnutrition and Food Habits* (Report of an International and Interprofessional Conference, Cuernavaca, Mexico, 1960). London.

484 FELIX, R. H. *et al.* 1961. *Mental Health and Social Welfare.* New York.

485 MEERLOO, J. A. M. 1952. 'Contribution of the psychiatrist to the management of crisis situations.' *Amer. J. Psychiat.* **109**: 352–5.

486 OPLER, M. K. (ed.) 1959. *Culture and Mental Health: Cross-cultural Studies.* New York.

487 PETRULLO, L. & BASS, B. M. (eds.) 1961. *Leadership and Interpersonal Behavior.* New York.

488 RUBIN, V. (ed.) 1960. *Culture, Society and Health.* New York.

489 WELFORD, A. T. *et al.* (eds.) 1962. *Society: Problems and Methods of Study.* London.

490 JOSIAH MACY, JR FOUNDATION. 1950. *Health and Human Relations in Germany.* New York.

491 JOSIAH MACY, JR FOUNDATION. 1951. *Health and Human Relations in Germany.* New York.

492 *Research into Factors Influencing Human Relations: Report of the International Conference (Nijmegen).* Hilversum, 1956.

493 WFMH. 1959. *Africa: Social Change and Mental Health – Report of a Panel Discussion. . . .* (New York, 23 March 1959). London.

Cultural Studies

494 BIESHEUVEL, S. 1960. 'Select bibliography on the aptitude of the African south of the Sahara, 1917–1958.' In *Mental*

Disorders and Mental Health in Africa South of the Sahara, CCTA/CSA Publ. No. 35. London. Pp. 263–9.

495 CAROTHERS, J. C. 1953. *The African Mind in Health and Disease: A Study in Ethnopsychiatry* (World Hlth Org. Monogr. Ser. 17). Geneva.

496 DUBOIS, J. A. 1906. *Hindu Manners, Customs and Ceremonies* (transl. from the French MS (1806) and ed. H. K. Beauchamp). (3rd ed.) Oxford. Pp. 160, 522–41.

497 GEBER, M. & DEAN, R. F. A. 1958. 'Psychomotor development in African children: The effects of social class and the need for improved tests.' *Bull. World Hlth Org.* **18**: 471–6.

498 HOFFET, F. 1951. *Psychanalyse de l'Alsace*. Paris.

499 HSU, F. L. K. (ed.) 1961. *Psychological Anthropology: Approaches to Culture and Personality*. Homewood, Illinois.

500 HUGHES, C. C. 1960. *An Eskimo Village in the Modern World*. Ithaca, N.Y.

501 KAPLAN, B. (ed.) 1961. *Studying Personality Cross-culturally*. New York.

502 LA BARRE, W. 1962. *They shall take up Serpents: Psychology of the Southern Snake-handling Cult*. Minneapolis. P. 160.

503 LIPSET, S. M. & LOWENTHAL, L. (eds.) 1961. *Culture and Social Character: The Work of David Riesman Reviewed*. New York.

504 MEAD, M. (ed.) 1953. *Cultural Patterns and Technical Change*. UNESCO, Paris.

505 MEAD, M. 1956. *New Lives for Old: Cultural Transformation – Manus, 1928–1953*. London.

506 MEAD, M. 1959. *An Anthropologist at Work: Writings of Ruth Benedict*. Boston.

507 MEAD, M. & WOLFENSTEIN, M. (eds.) 1955 & 1962. *Childhood in Contemporary Cultures*. Chicago.

508 MEADE, J. E. *et al.* 1961. *The Economic and Social Structure of Mauritius*. London.

509 OPLER, M. K. 1956. 'Ethnic differences in behaviour and psychopathology: Italian and Irish.' *Int. J. soc. Psychiat.* **2**: 11–22.

510 SODDY, K. (ed.) 1955–56. *Mental Health and Infant Development* (Proc. WFMH Int. Seminar, Chichester, 1952). Vol. 1: *Papers and Discussions*; Vol. 2: *Case Histories*. 2 vols. London & New York.

511 WAGLEY, C. (ed.) 1952. *Race and Class in Rural Brazil*. UNESCO, Paris.

512 CCTA/CSA. 1960. *CSA Meeting of Specialists on the Basic Psychology of African and Madagascan Populations* (Tananarive, 1959). Publ. No. 51. London.

SOME SOCIAL QUESTIONS

I. *Ageing*

513 TIBBITTS, C. (ed.) 1960. *Handbook of Social Gerontology: Social Aspects of Aging*. Chicago.

514 TIBBITTS, C. & DONAHUE, W. (eds.) 1960. *Aging in Today's Society*. New Jersey.

515 TOWNSEND, P. 1959. 'Social surveys of old age in Great Britain 1945–58.' *Bull. World Hlth Org.* **21**: 583–91.

II. *Industrialization and Urbanization*

516 CLAY, H. M. 1960. *The Older Worker and his Job* (Problems of Progress in Industry, No. 7). London.

517 CROOME, H. 1960. *Human Problems of Innovation* (Problems of Progress in Industry, No. 5). London.

518 FRIEDMAN, G. 1955. *Industrial Society: The Emergence of the Human Problems of Automation*. Glencoe, Ill.

519 RODGER, A. 1959. 'Ten years of ergonomics.' *Nature, Lond.*, **184**: 20–2.

520 SCOTT, J. F. & LYNTON, R. P. 1952. *The Community Factor in Modern Technology*. UNESCO, Paris.

521 THOMSON, D. C. (ed.) 1957. *Management, Labour and Community*, London.

522 VEIL, C. 1957. 'Phénóménologie du travail.' *Evolut. psychiat.* **4**: 693–721.

523 WELFORD, A. T. 1960. *Ergonomics of Automation* (Problems of Progress in Industry, No. 8). London.

524 CARNEGIE STUDY GROUP. 1958. 'Proceedings of the Carnegie Study Group on the basic principles of automation (Geneva, 1957).' *Int. soc. Sci. Bull.* **10**: 1.

525 ILO. 1961. 'Ergonomics: The scientific approach to making work human.' *Int. Labour Rev.* **83**: 1–35.

526 UNESCO. 1956. *The Social Implications of Industrialization and Urbanization in Africa South of the Sahara.* Paris.

527 UNESCO. 1956. *The Social Implications of Industrialization and Urbanization: Five Studies of Urban Populations of Recent Rural Origin in Cities of Southern Asia.* Calcutta.

528 UNITED KINGDOM. 1956. *Automation: A Report on the Technical Trends and their Impact on Management and Labour.* Dept Sci. Industr. Res., London.

529 UNITED KINGDOM. 1957. *Men, Steel and Technical Change* (Problems of Progress in Industry, No. 1). London.

530 UNITED KINGDOM. 1960. *Woman, Wife and Worker* (Problems of Progress in Industry, No. 10). London.

531 WFMH. 1957. *Mental Health Aspects of Urbanisation* (Report of discussions conducted in the Economic & Social Council Chamber, United Nations, New York, 1957, by WFMH). London.

532 WHO. 1958. Mental Health Aspects of the Peaceful Uses of Atomic Energy: Report of a Study Group. *World Hlth Org. tech. Rep. Ser.* 151. Geneva.

533 WHO. 1960. 'The psycho-social environment in industry.' *World Hlth Org. Chron.* **14**: 276–9.

III. *International Action*

534 BERGER, G. *et al.* 1959. 'Rapports de l'Occident avec le reste du monde.' *Perspectives*, Paris, No. 3 (avril). (Cf. English review: *World ment. Hlth* 1959, **11**: 190–5.)

535 KISKER, G. W. (ed.) 1951. *World Tensions: The Psychopathology of International Relations.* New York.

536 OPLER, M. E. 1954. *Social Aspects of Technical Assistance in Operation*. UNESCO, Paris.

537 UNESCO. 1953. *Interrelations of Cultures: Their Contribution to International Understanding*. Paris.

538 UNESCO. 1957. *The Nature of Conflict: Studies on the Sociological Aspects of International Tensions*. Paris.

539 WFMH. 1955. *Social Implications of Technical Assistance* (Report of a meeting held at the UN, New York, 1955). London.

IV. *Migration and Social Displacement*

540 BORRIE, W. D. *et al.* 1959. *The Cultural Integration of Immigrants*. UNESCO, Paris.

541 CURLE, A. & TRIST, E. 1947. 'Transitional communities and social reconnection.' *Human Relations* **1**: 42–68, 240–288.

542 MURPHY, H. B. M. *et al.* 1955. *Flight and Resettlement*. UNESCO, Paris.

543 ILO. 1959. *International Migration, 1945–1957* (Studies and Reports, No. 54). Geneva.

544 ILO. 1961. 'Some aspects of the international migration of families.' *Int. Labour Rev.* **83**: 65–86.

545 WFMH. 1960. *Uprooting and Resettlement* (11th Ann. Meeting WFMH, Vienna, 1958). London.

V. *Population*

546 LORIMER, F. *et al.* 1954. *Culture and Human Fertility*. UNESCO, Paris.

547 PINCUS, G. 1961. 'Suppression of ovulation with reference to oral contraceptives.' In *Modern Trends in Endocrinology*, 2nd ser., ed. H. Gardiner-Hill. London. Pp. 231–45.

548 TITMUSS, R. M. & ABEL SMITH, B. 1961. *Social Policies and Population Growth in Mauritius*. London.

549 'Mauritius and Malthus.' 1961. *Lancet* **1**: 542–3.

550 UNITED KINGDOM. 1960. *Report of the Departmental Committee on Human Artificial Insemination.* Home Office & Scottish Home Dept, London.

SOME SOCIAL DIFFICULTIES

I. *Delinquency*

551 ERIKSON, E. H. 1956. *New Perspectives for Research on Juvenile Delinquency.* Washington, D.C.

552 WILKINS, L. T. 1960. *Delinquent Generations.* London.

553 UN DEPT. OF ECON. SOCIAL AFFAIRS (DIV. OF SOCIAL WELFARE). 1952–58. *Comparative Survey on Juvenile Delinquency.* Pt I: North America (revised ed.); Pt II: Europe (in French*); Pt III: Latin America (revised ed.) (in Spanish**); Pt IV: Asia and the Far East; Pt V: Middle East. New York.
(*English summary in *Int. Rev. crim. Policy*, 1954, No. 5: 19–38.)
(**Cf. also J. A. Smythe, 'Juvenile delinquency in Latin American countries.' *Int. Rev. crim. Policy*, 1954, No. 5: 9–18.)

II. *Pathological Attitudes and Mental Disorder*

554 CARSTAIRS, G. M. 1958. 'Some problems of psychiatry in patients from alien cultures.' *Lancet* **1**: 1217–20.

555 EISLER, R. 1951. *Man into Wolf: An Anthropological Interpretation of Sadism, Masochism and Lycanthropy.* London.

556 FIELD, M. J. 1955. 'Witchcraft as a primitive interpretation of mental disorder.' *J. ment. Sci.* **101**: 826–33.
(Cf. also *J. ment. Sci.* **108**: 1043.)

557 GILLIS, L. 1962. *Human Behaviour in Illness: Psychology and Interpersonal Relationships.* With a contribution by S. Biesheuvel. London.

558 JUNG, C. G. 1959. *Flying Saucers: A Modern Myth of Things seen in the Skies* (transl. R. F. C. Hull). London.

559 MEERLOO, J. A. M. 1957. *Mental Seduction and Menticide: The Psychology of Thought Control and Brainwashing.* London.

560 MEERLOO, J. A. M. 1958. '"Infection mentale": Communication archaïque et régression insensible – Contribution à l'étude psychosomatique des épidémies mentales.' *Méd. et Hyg., Genève,* **16**: 469 et seq.

561 MEERLOO, J. A. M. 1958. 'The delusion of the flying saucer.' *Amer. Practitioner* **9**: 1631–6.

562 MEERLOO, J. A. M. 1959. 'Rock 'n roll: A modern aspect of St Vitus dance – implications for the theory of mental contagion.' *Amer. Practitioner* **10**: 1029–32.

563 SARGANT, W. 1957. *Battle for the Mind: A Physiology of Conversion and Brain-Washing.* London.

564 STENGEL, E. & COOK, N. G. 1958. *Attempted Suicide: Its Social Significance and Effects* (Maudsley Monogr. No. 4). London.

565 WITTKOWER, E. D. & FRIED, J. 1959. 'A cross-cultural approach to mental health problems.' *Amer. J. Psychiat.* **116**: 423–8.

566 CHURCH [OF ENGLAND] ASSEMBLY BOARD FOR SOCIAL RESPONSIBILITY. 1959. *Ought Suicide to be a Crime? – A Discussion of Suicide, Attempted Suicide and the Law.* London.

567 MILBANK MEMORIAL FUND. 1953. *Interrelations between the Social Environment and Psychiatric Disorders.* New York.

III. *Prejudice and Discrimination*

568 ADORNO, T. W. *et al.* 1950. *The Authoritarian Personality.* New York.

569 ALLPORT, G. W. 1954. *The Nature of Prejudice.* Cambridge, Mass.

570 BIESHEUVEL, S. 1959. *Race, Culture and Personality.* Johannesburg.

571 MYERS, J. K. & ROBERTS, B. 1959. *Family and Class Dynamics*. London.

572 GROUP FOR THE ADVANCEMENT OF PSYCHIATRY (GAP). 1957. *Psychological Aspects of School Desegregation* (Report No. 37). New York.

573 UNESCO. 1956. *The Race Question in Modern Science*. Paris.

IV. *Problems of Sex Behaviour*

574 ALLEN, C. 1958. *Homosexuality: Its Nature, Causation and Treatment*. London. (Cf. especially Pt. III: 'Social Significance'; pp. 54–63.)

575 BAILEY, D. S. (ed.) 1956. *Sexual Offenders and Social Punishment*. Church of England Moral Welfare Council, London.

576 FORD, C. S. & BEACH, F. A. 1951. *Patterns of Sexual Behavior*. New York.

577 WESTWOOD, G. 1960. *A Minority: A Report of the Life of the Male Homosexual in Great Britain*. London.

578 BRITISH MEDICAL ASS. 1955. *Homosexuality and Prostitution*. London.

579 UNITED KINGDOM. 1957. *Report of the Committee on Homosexual Offences and Prostitution*. Home Office, Scottish Home Dept, London.

Professional Training

PSYCHIATRY AND THE MEDICAL UNDERGRADUATE

580 BALINT, M. 1961. 'The pyramid and the psychotherapeutic relationship.' (Re: Training of medical students.) *Lancet* **2**: 1051–4.

581 BARTON HALL, S., HEARNSHAW, L. S. & HETHERINGTON, R. R. 1961. 'The teaching of psychology in the medical curriculum.' *J. ment. Sci.* **107**: 1003–10.

582 CURRAN, D. 1955. 'The place of psychology and psychiatry in medical education.' *Brit. med. J.* **2**: 515–18.

583 HARGREAVES, G. R., BROWN, D. G. & WHYTE, M. B. H. 1962. 'Home visits by medical students: An aspect of psychiatric education.' *Lancet* **2**: 141–2.

584 HENDERSON, D. 1955. 'Why psychiatry?' *Brit. med. J.* **2**: 519–23.

585 HILL, D. 1960. 'Acceptance of psychiatry by the medical student.' *Brit. med. J.* **1**: 917–18.

586 LEVINE, M. & LEDERER, H. D. 1959. 'Teaching of psychiatry in medical schools.' In *American Handbook of Psychiatry*, ed. S. Arieti. New York. Vol. 2: 1923–34.

587 MACCALMAN, D. R. 1953. 'Observations on the teaching of the principles of mental health to medical students' (and Memorandum on undergraduate teaching of psychiatry – from the Roy. Med.-Psychol. Ass.). *Brit. J. med. Psychol.* **26**: 140–51.

588 PARKER, S. 1960. 'The attitudes of medical students toward their patients: An exploratory study.' *J. med. Educ.* **35**: 849–56.

589 RICKLES, N. K. 1960. 'General medicine before specialization.' *Amer. J. Psychiat.* **116**: 663.

590 STEVENSON, I. 1961. *Medical History-taking*. New York.

591 TANNER, J. M. 1958. 'The place of human biology in medical education.' *Lancet* **1**: 1185–8.

592 TREDGOLD, R. F. 1962. 'The integration of psychiatric teaching into the curriculum.' *Lancet* 1. 1344–7.

593 AMERICAN PSYCHIATRIC ASS. 1952. *Psychiatry and Medical Education.* Washington, D.C.

594 'Psychological medicine and undergraduate education.' 1958. *Brit. med. J.* **2**: 602.

595 WHO. 1961. The Undergraduate Teaching of Psychiatry and Mental Health Promotion: 9th Report of the Expert Committee on Mental Health. *World Hlth Org. tech. Rep. Ser.* 208. Geneva.

596 WHO. 1961. *Teaching of Psychiatry and Mental Health* (World Hlth Org. publ. Hlth Papers 9). Geneva.

PSYCHIATRY AND THE MEDICAL POSTGRADUATE

597 BLEULER, M. *et al.* 1961. *Teaching of Psychiatry and Mental Health* (World Hlth Org. publ. Hlth Papers 9). Geneva.

598 DAVIES, T. T., DAVIES, E. T. L. & O'NEILL, D. 1958. 'Case-work in the teaching of psychiatry.' *Lancet* **2**: 34–7.

599 GILDEA, E. F. 1959. 'Teaching of psychiatry to residents.' In *American Handbook of Psychiatry*, ed. S. Arieti. New York. Vol. 2: 1935–47.

600 HOLT, R. R. & LUBORSKY, L. 1958. *Personality Patterns of Psychiatrists: A Study of Methods of Selecting Residents.* New York.

601 LEVY, D. M. 1959. *The Demonstration Clinic for the Psychological Study and Treatment of Mother and Child in Medical Practice.* Springfield, Ill.

602 MEARES, A. 1960. 'Communication with the patient.' *Lancet* **1**: 663–7.

603 AMERICAN PSYCHIATRIC ASS. 1953. *The Psychiatrist: His Training and Development.* Washington, D.C.

604 ROYAL MEDICO-PSYCHOL. ASS. 1951. *Memorandum on the Training of the Consultant Child Psychiatrist.* London.

605 ROYAL MEDICO-PSYCHOL. ASS. 1960. *The Recruitment and Training of the Child Psychiatrist.* London.

(Cf. Recruitment and training of child psychiatrists. *Brit. med. J.*, 1960. **2**: 205–6.)

PSYCHIATRY AND THE GENERAL PRACTITIONER

606 BALINT, M. 1954. 'Training general practitioners in psychotherapy.' *Brit. med. J.* **1**: 115–20.

607 CARSTAIRS, G. M., WALTON, H. J. & FAWCETT, P. G. 1962. 'General practitioners and psychological medicine: Their views on a postgraduate course.' *Lancet* **2**: 397.

608 GOSHEN, C. E. 1959. 'A project for the creation of better understanding of psychiatry by the general practitioner.' *Southern med. J.* **52**: 30–4.

OTHER PROFESSIONAL TRAINING IN THE MENTAL HEALTH FIELD

609 AFFLECK, J. W. *et al.* 1960. 'In-service mental-health teaching for health visitors.' *Lancet* **2**: 641–3.

610 CAPLAN, G. 1959. 'An approach to the education of community mental health specialists.' *Ment. Hyg.* **43**: 268–80.

611 FERARD, M. L. & HUNNYBUN, N. K. 1962. *The Caseworker's Use of Relationships.* London.

612 JAMES, E. 1958. 'The education of the scientist.' *Brit. med. J.* **2**: 575–6.

613 WRIGHT, M. S. 1962. *An Interim Report on the Characteristics of Successful and Unsuccessful Student Nurses in Scotland.* Edinburgh.
(*As summarized:* Intelligence and student nurses. *Brit. med. J.*, 1962, **2**: 37–8.)

614 AMERICAN ASS. PSYCHIAT. SOCIAL WORKERS. 1950. *Education for Psychiatric Social Work.* New York.

615 (BRITISH) ASS. PSYCHIAT. SOCIAL WORKERS. 1957. *Essentials of Case Work.* London.

616 ENGLAND & WALES. 1962. *The Training of Staff of Training Centres for the Mentally Subnormal.* Ministry of Health

(Central Health Services Council Standing Mental Health Advisory Committee), London.
617 LEVERHULME STUDY GROUP. 1961. *The Complete Scientist: An Inquiry into the Problem of achieving Breadth in the Education at School and University of Scientists, Engineers and other Technologists* (Report of the Leverhulme Study Group to the Brit. Ass. Advance. Sci.). London.
618 'Papers on the Teaching of Personality Development.' 1958. *Sociol. Rev. Monogr.* No. 1.
619 WFMH. 1956. *Mental Health in Teacher Education.* London.
620 WHO. 1956. Expert Committee on Psychiatric Nursing: 1st Report. *World Hlth Org. tech. Rep. Ser.* 105. Geneva.

AUDIO-VISUAL AIDS

621 PILKINGTON, T. L. 1960. 'The use of film in psychiatry.' *World ment. Hlth* **12**: 143–5.
622 RUHE, D. S. *et al.* 1960. 'Television in the teaching of psychiatry: Report of four years' preliminary development.' *J. med. Educ.* **35**: 916–26.
623 STAFFORD-CLARK, D. *et al.* 1961. 'Television in medical education.' *Brit. med. J.* **1**: 500.

CATALOGUES OF FILMS FOR PSYCHIATRIC, PROFESSIONAL, AND PUBLIC EDUCATION:

624 (*a*) Deutsches Zentralinstitut für Lehrmittel. 1960. *Verzeichnis der wissenschaftlichen Filme.* Berlin (East Germany).
625 (*b*) Institut für der wissenschaftlichen Filme. 1960. *Gesamtverzeichnis der wissenschaftlichen Filme.* Göttingen (German Federal Republic).
626 (*c*) La Presse Médicale. 1956–57. *Films médicaux et chirurgicaux français*, ed. P. Détrie. Paris, 1956; Supplément, 1957.
627 (*d*) Scientific Film Ass. 1960. *Films of Psychology and Psychiatry.* London.

628 (*e*) U.S. Information Agency. 1956. *United States Educational, Scientific, and Cultural Motion Pictures and Filmstrips: Science Section*. Washington, D.C.

629 (*f*) WFMH. 1960. *International Catalogue of Mental Health Films*, ed. T. L. Pilkington. (2nd ed.) London.

Public Education in Mental Health

PROGRAMMES AND THEIR EVALUATION

630 MEAD, M. 1959. 'Cultural factors in community-education programs.' In *Community Education Principles and Practices from World-wide Experience* (58th Yearbook of the Nat. Soc. for the Study of Education), ed. N. B. Henry. Chicago.

631 POWELL, E. 1961. Everybody's business: Emerging patterns for mental health services and the public (NAMH London Ann. Conf.). As reported in *Brit. med. J.* **1**: 820. (Cf. *Lancet* **1**: 608–9.)

632 RIDENOUR, N. 1953. 'Criteria of effectiveness in mental health education.' *Amer. J. Orthopsychiat.* **23**: 271–9.

633 PENNSYLVANIA MENTAL HEALTH, INC. 1960. *Mental Health Education: A Critique.* Philadelphia.

634 WHO. 1958. Expert Committee on Training of Health Personnel in Health Education of the Public. *World Hlth Org. tech. Rep. Ser.* 156. Geneva.

635 WHO. 1959. Conference on Mental Hygiene Practice (Helsinki, 1959). Report of Committee C: The Education of the Public in Mental Health Principles. WHO Regional Office for Europe, Copenhagen. (Duplicated document.)

PROGRAMMES FOR PARENTS

636 ISAMBERT, A. 1960. *L'Education des parents.* Paris.

637 ISAMBERT, A. 1960. 'Parent education in France.' *World ment. Hlth* **12**: 130–3.

638 LEWIS, R. S., STRAUSS, A. A. & LEHTINEN, L. E. 1960. *The Brain-Injured Child: A Book for Parents and Laymen.* (2nd ed.) London.

639 MACKAY, J. L. 1960. 'Parent education in the United States of America.' *World ment. Hlth* **12**: 76–85.

640 STERN, H. H. 1960. *Parent Education: An International Survey*. Univ. of Hull, & UNESCO Inst. for Education. Hull.

641 LOUISIANA ASS. MENTAL HEALTH. 1957. *The New Revised and Extended 'Pierre the Pelican' Series*. 28 issues. New Orleans.

Popular Concepts of Mental Health

642 CARSTAIRS, G. M. & WING, J. K. 1958. 'Attitudes of the general public to mental illness.' *Brit. med. J.* **2**: 594–7.

643 LEMKAU, P. V. & CROCETTI, G. M. 1962. 'An urban population's opinion and knowledge about mental illness.' *Amer. J. Psychiat.* **118**: 692–700.

644 NUNNALLY, J. C., JR. 1961. *Popular Conceptions of Mental Health: Their Development and Change*. New York.

645 PAUL, B. D. (ed.) 1955. *Health, Culture and Community: Case Studies of Public Reactions to Health Programs*. New York.

Use of the Mass Media

646 ESSEX-LOPRESTI, M. 1961. 'National television programmes.' *Med. biol. Illustr.* **11**: 68.

647 JACOBY, A. 1960. 'On using mental health films.' In *International Catalogue of Mental Health Films*. (2nd ed.) WFMH, London. Pp. 6–7.

648 AMERICAN PSYCHIATRIC ASS. 1956. *Psychiatry, The Press and the Public: Problems in Communication*. Washington, D.C.

649 WHO. 1959. *World Health* **12**, No. 3 (May–June 1959). Special issue: Mental Health.

650 WHO. 1961. *World Health* **14**, No. 4 (July–Aug. 1961). To counter mental illness: Science. A special issue to mark the conclusion of the Mental Health Year (1960–61).

Additional References

651 KAY, D. & ROTH, M. 1961. 'Physical disability and emotional factors in the mental disorders.' Paper read at the IIIrd World Congress of Psychiatry, Montreal, June 1961.

652 SELLIN, T. 1938. 'Culture conflict and crime.' *Soc. Sci. Res. Bull.* **41**; *Am. J. Sociol.* **44**: 97–103.

653 BOWLBY, J. 1960. 'Grief and mourning in infancy and early childhood.' *Psycho-Anal. Study Child* **15**: 9–52.

654 BOWLBY, J. 1961. 'Processes of mourning.' *Int. J. Psycho-Anal.* **42**: 317–40.

655 BOWLBY, J. 1961. 'Childhood mourning and its implications for psychiatry.' *Am. J. Psychiat.* **118**: 481.

656 BUCKLE, D. F. 1962. 'Quelques aspects de l'évolution de la pratique psychiatrique en Europe.' *L'information psychiatrique* **5**: No. 5.

(in English: 'Some developments of psychiatric practice in Europe.' 1962. *Aust. Psychiat. Bull.* **3**: Nos. 3 & 4.

in Czech: 'K Vyvoji psychiatrické praxe v Evrope.' 1963. *Cs. Psychiat.* **59**.

in Greek: 'Exelixis tinés ton efarmogon tis psykiatrikis is tin Evropin.' *Arch. med. Sci.*, Athens, 1962, No. 2.)

657 ZIER, A. & DOSHAY, L. J. 1957. 'Procyclidine hydrochloride ("Kemadrin") treatment of parkinsonism.' *Neurology* **7**: 485–9.

658 SCHWAB, R. S. 1959. 'Problems in the treatment of Parkinson's disease in elderly patients.' *Geriatrics* **14**: 545–58.

659 LINDSAY, T. F. 1961. 'When scientists stop being human.' *Daily Telegraph*, London, 19 January.

660 PENROSE, L. S. 1959. 'The somatic chromosomes in mongolism.' *Lancet* **1**: 710.

661 KORZYBSKI. 1927. *Science and Sanity*.

662 KORZYBSKI. 1931. *Un système non-aristotélien et sa nécessité pour la rigeur en mathématique et en physique*. Communication to the Congress of the American Mathematical Society, New Orleans.

663 MOUNIER, E. 1949. *Le personnalisme*. Paris. Pp. 8–10. (English transl. *Personalism*. London, 1952.)

664 JAQUES, E. 1951. *The Changing Culture of a Factory*. London.

665 PASAMANICK, B. & LILIENFELD, A. M. 1955. 'The association of maternal and foetal factors with the development of mental deficiency.' *J.A.M.A.* **159**: 155–60.

666 STAR, SHIRLEY. 1952. *Attitudes to Mental Illness*. Chicago: National Opinion Research Center Study. (Mimeographed.)

667 RIESMAN, D. 1950. *The Lonely Crowd*. New Haven.

668 MAIN, T. F. 1958. 'Some thoughts on group behaviour.' Paper read at the Davidson Clinic Summer School, Edinburgh, 1958. (Unpublished.)

669 SIGERIST, H. E. 1945. *Civilization and Disease*. New York. Pp. 66–71.

670 CURRAN, D. 1952. 'Psychiatry Ltd.' *J. ment. Sci.* **98**: 373–81.

671 TREDGOLD, R. F. & SODDY, K. 1963. *Tredgold's Textbook of Mental Deficiency*. (10th edition.) London. Pp. 98 and 151–229.

672 MIDDENDORF, W. 1960. *New Forms of Juvenile Delinquency: their Origin, Prevention and Treatment* (2nd UN Congress Prev. Crime & Treat. Offenders). UN Dept. Econ. Social Affairs, New York.

673 LEBOVICI, S. 1959. 'La prévention en santé mentale chez l'enfant.' Réflexions à propos du Seminar de Copenhague sous les auspices de l'Organisation mondiale de la Santé, 1958. *Psychiatrie de l'Enfant* **2**: 197–226.

674 ENGEL, G. L. 1961. 'Is grief a disease?' *Psychosomat. Med.* **23**: 18–22.

675 SPITZ, R. 1945. *The Psychoanalytic Study of the Child* **1**: 53. ibid. 1946, **2**: 113.

Supplementary Titles

ABRAMS, A., TOMAN, J. E. P. & GARNER, H. H. 1963. *Unfinished Tasks in the Behavioral Sciences*. London.

ALLINSMITH, W. & GOETHALS, G. W. 1962. *The Role of Schools in Mental Health*. New York.

APLEY, J. & MACKEITH, R. 1962. *The Child and his Symptoms*. Oxford.

ATKIN, I. 1962. *Aspects of Psychotherapy*. Edinburgh.

BARTON, WALTER. 1962. *Administration in Psychiatry*. Springfield, Illinois.

BOCKHOVEN, J. S. 1963. *Moral Treatment in American Psychiatry*. New York.

BOSCH, GERHARD. 1962. *Der Frühkindliche Autismus*. Berlin, Göttingen, Heidelberg.

CLARK, D. H. 1964. *Administrative Therapy*. London.

COHEN, JOHN. (ed.) 1964. *Readings in Psychology*. London.

CURRAN, D. & PARTRIDGE, M. 1963. *Psychological Medicine*. Edinburgh.

DAVIES, E. B. (ed.) 1964. *Depression* (Proceedings of a symposium by the Cambridge Postgraduate Medical School). London.

DUHL, L. J. (ed.) 1963. *The Urban Condition. People and Policy in the Metropolis*. New York.

EPSTEIN, C. 1962. *Intergroup Relations for Police Officers*. London.

FISH, F. J. 1963. *Clinical Psychiatry for the Layman*. Bristol.

FISH, F. J. 1964. *An Outline of Psychiatry for Students and Practitioners*. Bristol.

FREEMAN, H. E. & SIMMONS, O. G. 1963. *The Mental Patient comes Home*. New York.

GETZELS, J. W. & JACKSON, P. W. 1962. *Creativity and Intelligence: Explorations with Gifted Students*. New York.

GIBSON, J. 1962. *Psychiatry for Nurses*. Oxford.

GIBSON, J. 1963. *A Guide to Psychiatry*. Oxford.
GILBERT, J. B. 1962. *Disease and Destiny*. London.
GOLDFARB, W. 1961. *Childhood Schizophrenia*. Cambridge, Mass.
HALLAS, C. H. 1962. *Nursing the Mentally Subnormal*. Bristol.
HEATON-WARD, W. A. 1963. *Mental Subnormality*. (2nd ed.) Bristol.
HOLMES, D. J. 1963. *The Adolescent in Psychotherapy*. London.
HOWELLS, J. G. 1963. *Family Psychiatry*. Edinburgh.
ILLINGWORTH, R. S. 1963. *The Normal School Child: His Problems, Physical and Emotional*. London.
JOHN, A. L. 1961. *A Study of the Psychiatric Nurse*. Edinburgh.
JOHNSTON, N., SAVITZ, L. & WOLFGANG, M. E. (eds.) 1962. *The Sociology of Punishment and Correction: A Book of Readings*. New York.
JONES, M. 1962. *Social Psychiatry: in the Community, in Hospitals and in Prisons*. Springfield, Illinois.
KAPLAN, M. 1960. *Leisure in America: a social inquiry*. New York.
KELLNER, R. 1963. *Family Ill Health*. London.
KRAKOWSKI, A. J. & SANTORA, D. A. 1962. *Child Psychiatry and the General Practitioner*. Illinois.
KRAMER, B. M. 1962. *Day Hospital*. New York.
LEIGHTON, A. H. *et al.* 1963. *Psychiatric Disorder among the Yoruba*. New York.
LIN, TSUNG-YI & STANDLEY, C. C. 1962. *The Scope of Epidimiology in Psychiatry* (World Hlth Org. publ. Hlth Papers 16). Geneva.
MACKENZIE, M. 1963. *Psychological Depression: A Common Disorder of Personality*. London.
MADDISON, D. C. 1963. *Psychiatric Nursing*. Edinburgh.
MARKS, P. A. & SEEMAN, W. 1963. *The Actuarial Description of Abnormal Personality*. London.
MCGHIE, A. 1963. *Psychology as applied to Nursing*. Edinburgh.
MOWBRAY, R. M. & RODGER, T. F. 1963. *Psychology in relation to Medicine*. Edinburgh.
OLMSTEAD, C. 1962. *Heads I win, Tails you lose*. New York.

PRONKO, N. H. 1963. *Textbook of Abnormal Psychology*. London.

PUGH, T. F. 1962. *Epidemiologic Findings in United States Mental Hospital Data*. London.

RICHTER, D., TANNER, J. M., TAYLOR, LORD & ZANGWILL, O. L. (eds.) 1962. *Aspects of Psychiatric Research*. London.

RIDENOUR, NINA. 1961. *Mental Health in the United States*. Harvard.

RODGER, T. F., INGRAM, I. M. & MOWBRAY, R. M. 1962. *Lecture Notes on Psychological Medicine*. Edinburgh.

SARGANT, W. & SLATER, E. 1963. *An Introduction to Physical Methods of Treatment in Psychiatry*. Edinburgh.

SARASON, S., DAVIDSON, K. & BLATT, B. 1962. *The Preparation of Teachers*. New York.

SCHIMEL, J. L. 1961. *How to be an Adolescent – and Survive*. New York.

SIM, M. 1963. *Guide to Psychiatry*. Edinburgh.

STAFFORD-CLARK, D. 1964. *Psychiatry for Students*. London.

STEINFELD, J. I. 1963. *A New Approach to Schizophrenia*. London.

TAYLOR, LORD & CHAVE, S. 1964. *Mental Health and Environment*. London.

THOMPSON, G. G. 1962. *Child Psychology*. London.

VALENTINE, M. *An Introduction to Psychiatry*. Edinburgh.

WAHL, C. W. 1963. *Psychosomatic Medicine*. London.

WEINBERG, A. A. 1961. *Migration and Belonging. A Study of Mental Health and Personal Adjustment in Israel*. The Hague.

WELFORD, A. T., ARGYLE, M., GLASS, D. V. & MORRIS, J. N. (eds.) 1962. *Society: Problems and Methods of Study*. New York.

WENAR, C., HANDLON, M. W. & GARNER, A. M. 1962. *Psychosomatic and Emotional Disturbances: A Study of Mother-Child-Relationships* (A Psychosomatic Medicine Monograph). New York.

WOLFGANG, M. E., SAVITZ, L. & JOHNSTON, N. (eds.) 1962. *The Sociology of Crime and Delinquency: a Book of Readings*. New York.

ZILBOORG, G. 1962. *Psychoanalysis and Religion.* New York.

VAN ZONNEVELD, R. J. 1961. *The Health of the Aged.* Edinburgh.

ASSOCIATION OF THE BAR OF THE CITY OF NEW YORK WITH CORNELL UNIVERSITY LAW SCHOOL. 1962. *Mental Illness and Due Process.* New York.

GROUP FOR THE ADVANCEMENT OF PSYCHIATRY (GAP), COMMITTEE ON HOSPITALS. 1963. *Public Relations: A Responsibility of the Mental Hospital Administration.* New York.

Proceedings of the Third World Congress of Psychiatry, Montreal. 1961. Vols I & II. Toronto and Montreal.

ROYAL MEDICO-PSYCHOL. ASS. 1963. *Hallucinogenic Drugs and their Psychotherapeutic Use* (Proceedings of a Meeting of the Association, 1961). London.

SOCIETY FOR PSYCHOSOMATIC RESEARCH. *The Nature of Stress Disorder* (Report of 1958 conference). London.

Index

For Product Safety Concerns and Information please contact our EU
representative GPSR@taylorandfrancis.com
Taylor & Francis Verlag GmbH, Kaufingerstraße 24, 80331 München, Germany

www.ingramcontent.com/pod-product-compliance
Ingram Content Group UK Ltd.
Pitfield, Milton Keynes, MK11 3LW, UK
UKHW022110190926
475702UK00013B/1360
* 9 7 8 1 1 3 8 8 8 1 3 9 6 *